Renal and Metabolic Disorders

Pittsburgh Critical Care Medicine series

Continuous Renal Replacement Therapy
edited by John A. Kellum, Rinaldo Bellomo, and Claudio Ronco

Renal and Metabolic Disorders
edited by John A. Kellum and Jorge Cerdá

Mechanical Ventilation
edited by Jonathan Kreit

Emergency Department Critical Care .
edited by Donald Yealy and Clifton Callaway

Trauma Intensive Care
edited by Samuel Tisherman and Racquel Forsythe

Abdominal Organ Transplant Patients
edited by Ali Al-Khafaji

Infection and Sepsis
edited by Peter Linden

Pediatric Intensive Care
edited by Scott Watson and Ann Thompson

Cardiac Problems
edited by Thomas Smitherman

ICU Procedures
by Scott Gunn and Holt Murray

Renal and Metabolic Disorders

Edited by

John A. Kellum, MD

Professor and Vice-Chair
Department of Critical Care Medicine
University of Pittsburgh
Pittsburgh, PA

and

Jorge Cerdá, MD

Clinical Professor of Medicine
Department of Medicine
Division of Nephrology
Albany Medical College
Albany, NY

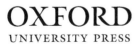
UNIVERSITY PRESS

OXFORD

UNIVERSITY PRESS

Oxford University Press is a department of the University of
Oxford. It furthers the University's objective of excellence
in research, scholarship, and education by publishing worldwide.

Oxford   New York
Auckland   Cape Town   Dar es Salaam   Hong Kong   Karachi
Kuala Lumpur   Madrid   Melbourne   Mexico City   Nairobi
New Delhi   Shanghai   Taipei   Toronto

With offices in
Argentina   Austria   Brazil   Chile   Czech Republic   France   Greece
Guatemala   Hungary   Italy   Japan   Poland   Portugal   Singapore
South Korea   Switzerland   Thailand   Turkey   Ukraine   Vietnam

Oxford is a registered trade mark of Oxford University Press in the UK
and certain other countries.

Published in the United States of America by
Oxford University Press
198 Madison Avenue, New York, NY 10016

Library of Congress Cataloging-in-Publication Data
Renal and metabolic disorders / edited by John A. Kellum and Jorge Cerdá.
   p. ; cm.—Pittsburgh critical care medicine series)
   Includes bibliographical references and index.
   ISBN 978-0-19-975160-0 (pbk. : alk. paper)
   I. Kellum, John A.   II. Cerdá, Jorge, 1949-   III. Series: Pittsburgh critical care medicine.
   [DNLM: 1. Kidney Diseases—therapy.   2. Critical Care.   3. Endocrine System
   Diseases—therapy.   4. Metabolic Diseases—-therapy. WJ 300]
   LC Classification not assigned
   616.6'106—dc23
   2012017048

9 8 7 6 5 4 3 2 1
printed in the United States of America
on acid-free paper

Dedication

We dedicate this volume to our ICU patients, their families and the nursing professionals caring for them, hoping we can all together make a difference in their lives.

Series Preface

No place in the world is more closely identified with Critical Care Medicine than Pittsburgh. In the late sixties, Peter Safar and Ake Grenvik pioneered the science and practice of critical care not just in Pittsburgh, but around the world. Their multidisciplinary team approach became the standard for how ICU care is delivered in Pittsburgh to this day. The Pittsburgh Critical Care Medicine series honors this tradition. Edited and largely authored by University of Pittsburgh faculty, the content reflects best practice in critical care medicine. The Pittsburgh model has been adopted by many programs around the world and local leaders are recognized as world leaders. It is our hope that through this series of concise handbooks a small part of this tradition can be passed on to the many practitioners of critical care the world over.

John A. Kellum
Series Editor

Preface

It is our pleasure to present this book to the wide audience of generalists, specialists, residents and medical students involved in the care of critically ill patients in the intensive care unit.

Our target is the colleague confronted with the intricacies of managing the metabolic and renal disturbances arising in such patients. We expect this book will help one recognize, understand and manage these conditions with fluency and confidence.

When critically ill patients develop acute kidney injury or severe, often life-threatening electrolyte and endocrine abnormalities, the complexity of the problem, the multiple interactions and the severe consequences of action or inaction make for a stressful situation. While standard textbooks are useful references, a quick review of basics afforded by slimmer texts is often needed particularly when the problem is both acute and unfamiliar.

Recognizing these circumstances, we have strived throughout the book to maintain a fluid, uncluttered format that makes quick consultation easy, and orients the hurried practitioner on how to take rapid, effective action.

We have endeavored to emphasize the interactions between processes and—at the risk of some repetition—have approached each chapter emphasizing the interplay between organ systems and metabolic processes.

The authors are all experts in their respective subjects, who are actually involved in the care of critically ill patients. We hope this book will allow a glimpse into the thought processes of these seasoned experts, and demonstrate their application of current knowledge in a rapidly evolving field.

We greatly appreciate the privilege of editing this book and hope it will be a useful tool in the management of these complex conditions.

John A Kellum and Jorge Cerdá
Spring, 2012

Contents

Contributors *xiii*

Section A: Renal Disease

1 AKI I: The critically ill patient — 1
2 Acute kidney injury in special circumstances — 11
3 AKI and sepsis — 23
4 The critically ill patient with chronic kidney disease — 29
5 Principles of fluid management — 39
6 Functional hemodynamic monitoring — 43
7 Pharmacologic therapy in acute kidney injury — 49
8 Drug dosing in kidney disease — 57
9 Renal replacement therapy (RRT) indications, timing, and patient selection — 69
10 Choosing a renal replacement therapy in acute kidney injury — 77
11 Combined kidney-lung failure — 91
12 Acute kidney injury in cirrhosis — 97
13 Renal disorders in pregnancy — 107
14 Renal disorders in pediatrics — 119
15 Acid-base disorders — 131
16 Electrolyte disorders — 137
17 Management of the renal transplant patient in the ICU — 143

Section B: Endocrine and Metabolic Disease

18 Diabetes mellitus — 159
19 Thyroid conditions in critical care — 171
20 Adrenal disease in critical care — 177
21 Calcium, bone, and mineral disease in the critically ill patient — 185
22 Nutrition in the critically ill patient — 201

Index   211

Contributors

Anjali Acharya

Division of Nephrology
Department of Medicine
Jacobi Medical Center
Albert Einstein College of Medicine
Bronx, NY

Sean M. Bagshaw

Division of Critical Care Medicine
University of Alberta Hospital
University of Alberta
Edmonton, Canada

Rinaldo Bellomo

Department of Intensive Care
Austin Hospital
Melbourne
Australia

Jodie Bryk

Chief Internal Medicine Resident
University of Pittsburgh Medical
    Center

Jorge Cerdá

Clinical Professor of Medicine
Department of Medicine
Division of Nephrology
Albany Medical College
Albany, NY

James Desemone

Director of Medical Staff Quality
    Ellis Medicine, Ellis Medicine,
    Schenectady, NY and
Clinical Associate Professor of
    Medicine
Albany Medical College
Albany, NY

Xaime García

Critical Care Department
Hospital of Sabadell-Autonomous
    University of Barcelona, Spain

Eric A.J. Hoste

Intensive Care Unit, Ghent University
    Hospital
Ghent University
Gent, Belgium and
Senior Clinical Investigator of the
    Research Foundation-Flanders
    (Belgium) (FWO)

Arun Jeyabalan

Associate Professor
Division of Maternal-Fetal Medicine
Dept of Obstetrics, Gynecology, and
    Reproductive Sciences
Magee-Womens Hospital
University of Pittsburgh School of
    Medicine
Pittsburgh, Pennsylvania

Belinda Jim

Division of Nephrology
Department of Medicine
Jacobi Medical Center
Albert Einstein College of Medicine
    Bronx, NY

John A. Kellum

Professor and Vice-Chair
Department of Critical Care
    Medicine
University of Pittsburgh
Pittsburgh, PA

Roy O. Mathew

Department of Medicine
Division of Nephrology
Albany Stratton VA Medical
    Center
Albany, NY

Jerry McCauley

Professor of Medicine, Department
    of Medicine
Professor of Surgery, Department
    of Surgery
Director, Transplant Nephrology,
    UPMC Transplantation
    Institute
Medical Director, Kidney/Pancreas
    Transplantation
University of Pittsburgh

Michael L. Moritz

Associate Professor, Pediatrics
Clinical Director, Pediatric
    Nephrology
Medical Director, Pediatric
    Dialysis
Children's Hospital of Pittsburgh
    at UPMC
University of Pittsburgh School
    of Medicine
Pittsburgh, PA

Mitra K. Nadim

Associate Professor of Clinical
    Medicine
Division of Nephrology
Department of Medicine
Keck School of Medicine of USC
University of Southern
    California

Christina Nguyen

Fellow, Pediatric Nephrology

Thomas D. Nolin

Assistant Professor
Center for Clinical Pharmaceutical
    Sciences and Department of
    Pharmacy and Therapeutics
School of Pharmacy and
Renal-Electrolyte Division
Department of Medicine
School of Medicine
University of Pittsburgh
Pittsburgh, PA

Juan Ochoa

Professor of Surgery and Critical
    Care
University of Pittsburgh
Medical and Scientific Director
Nestle Health Care Nutrition,
    Nestle Health Science
North America

Abhinetri Pandula

Internal Medicine, Stratton Veterans
    Administration Medical Center,
    Albany, NY
Instructor of Medicine, Albany
    Medical College

Neesh Pannu

Associate Professor of Medicine
Division of Nephrology
University of Alberta
Edmonton, Canada

Michael R. Pinsky

Vice-Chair, Academic Affairs
Professor of Critical Care Medicine,
    Bioengineering, Cardiovascular
    Disease and Anesthesiology
606 Scaife Hall
3550 Terrace Street
Pittsburgh, PA

Claudio Ronco
Director
Dep. Nephrology Dialysis &
 Transplantation
International Renal Research
 Institute (IRRIV)
San Bortolo Hospital
Vicenza, Italy

Kai Singbartl
Associate Professor
Department of Anesthesiology
Penn State College of Medicine
Milton S. Hershey Medical Center
Hershey, PA

Kristine S. Schonder
Assistant Professor
Department of Pharmacy and
 Therapeutics
School of Pharmacy
University of Pittsburgh and
Clinical Pharmacist
Ambulatory Care and Transplant
Thomas E. Starzl Transplantation
 Institute
University of Pittsburgh Medical Center
Pittsburgh, PA

Nirav Shah
Assistant Professor of Medicine
University of Pittsburgh

Shamik Shah
Critical Care & Transplant
 Nephrologist, Apollo Hospitals
Ahmedabad
India

Aditya Uppalapati
Assistant Professor of Medicine
St. Louis University, School of
 Medicine

Section A

Renal Disease

Chapter 1

AKI I: The critically ill patient

Aditya Uppalapati and John A. Kellum

The terms acute kidney injury (AKI) and acute renal failure are not synonymous. Although the term *renal failure* is best reserved for patients who have lost renal function to the point that life can no longer be sustained without intervention, AKI is used to describe patients with earlier or milder forms of acute renal dysfunction as well as those with overt failure. Although the analogy is imperfect, the AKI—renal failure relationship can be thought of as being similar to acute coronary syndrome and myocardial infarction with cardiogenic shock. AKI is intended to describe the entire spectrum of disease from relatively mild to severe. By contrast, renal failure is defined as renal function inadequate to clear the waste products of metabolism despite the absence of or correction of hemodynamic or mechanical causes. Clinical manifestations of renal failure (either acute or chronic) include:

- Uremic symptoms (drowsiness, nausea, hiccough, twitching)
- Hyperkalemia
- Hyponatremia
- Metabolic acidosis

Oliguria

Persistent oliguria may be a feature of acute renal failure but nonoliguric renal failure is not uncommon. Patients may continue to make urine despite an inadequate glomerular filtration. Although prognosis is often better if urine output is maintained, use of diuretics to promote urine output does not seem to improve outcome (and some studies even suggest harm).

Classification

International consensus criteria for AKI have been purposed. The acronym RIFLE is used to describe three levels of renal impairment (Risk, Injury, Failure) and two clinical outcomes (Loss and End-stage kidney disease).

The RIFLE classification system includes separate criteria for serum creatinine and urine output. The criteria, which lead to the worst classification, define the

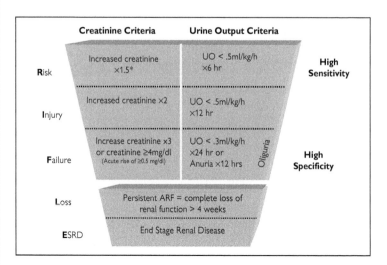

Figure 1.1 Modified RIFLE criteria for Acute Kidney Injury (AKI). Patients are diagnosed with AKI if they meet any criteria and then staged according to the most severe criterion.
*Recently "Risk" was expanded by the Acute Kidney Injury Network to include any increase in serum creatinine of at least 0.3 mg/dl, even if less than 50 percent increase, as long as it is documented to occur over 48 hrs or less..

stage of AKI. Note that RIFLE-F is present even if the increase in SCrt is < threefold, so long as the new SCrt is < 4.0 mg/dl in the setting of an acute increase of at least 0.5 mg/dl. The shape of the figure denotes the fact that more patients (high sensitivity) will be included in the mild category, including some without actually having renal failure (less specificity). In contrast, at the bottom, the criteria are strict and, therefore, specific, but some patients will be missed.

Incidence and progression

Acute Kidney Injury occurs in 35–65 percent of ICU admissions and 5–20 percent of general hospital admissions. Mortality rates increase significantly with AKI and most studies show a three- to fivefold increase in the risk of death in hospital with AKI compared to patients without AKI. Furthermore, increases in severity of AKI are associated with a stepwise increase in risk of death such that patients reaching RIFLE-F are far more likely to die prior to hospital discharge compared to patients that do not progress from RIFLE-R or RIFLE-I. Hospital mortality rates for ICU patients with AKI are approximately: R-9 percent, I-11 percent, F-26 percent compared to 6 percent for ICU patients without AKI. Unfortunately, more than 50 percent of patients with RIFLE-R progress to class I (in approximately 1–2 days) or F (in approximately 3–4 days) and almost 30 percent of RIFLE-I progress to F.

Risk factors for AKI

Risk factors for developing AKI as defined by RIFLE criteria:
- Sepsis.
- Increasing age, especially age >62 years.
- Race: Black patients for developing RIFLE-F.
- Greater severity of illness as per Acute Physiology and Chronic Health Evaluation III (APACHE III) or Sepsis-related Organ Failure Assessment (SOFA) scores.
- Preexisting chronic kidney disease.
- Prior admission to a non-ICU ward in the hospital.
- Surgical admissions more likely than medical admissions.
- Cardiovascular disease.
- Emergent surgeries.
- Patients on mechanical ventilators.

Etiology of AKI

Clinical features may suggest the cause of AKI and dictate further investigation. Acute kidney injury is common in the critically ill, especially in patients with sepsis and other forms of systemic inflammation (e.g., major surgery, trauma, burns) but other causes must be considered. In sepsis, the kidney often has a normal histological appearance.

Volume responsive AKI

It is estimated that as many as 50 percent of cases of AKI are "fluid responsive" and the first step in managing any case of AKI is to ensure appropriate fluid resuscitation. However, volume overload is a key factor contributing to the mortality attributable to AKI so ongoing fluid administration to non-fluid-responsive patients should be discouraged. In general, fluid resuscitation should be guided by hemodynamic monitoring.

Sepsis-induced AKI

Sepsis is a primary cause or contributing factor in more than 50 percent of cases of AKI including those cases severe enough to require renal replacement therapy (RRT). Patients with sepsis develop AKI at rates as high as 40 percent even when considering patients outside the ICU. Septic shock appears to be an important factor in the development of sepsis-induced AKI; however, patients without overt shock do not appear to be any less likely to develop AKI.

Hypotension

Hypotension is an important risk factor for AKI and many patients with AKI have sustained at least one episode hypotension. Treating fluid-responsive AKI with fluid resuscitation is clearly an important step, but many patients will also require vasoactive therapy (e.g., dopamine, norepinephrine) to maintain arterial blood pressure. Despite a common belief among many practitioners, norepinephrine does not increase the risk of AKI compared to dopamine, and in animals with sepsis, renal blood flow actually increases with norepinephrine.

Postoperative AKI

Risk factors include hypovolemia, hypotension, major abdominal surgery, and sepsis. Surgical procedures (particularly gynecological) may be complicated by damage to the lower urinary tract with an obstructive nephropathy. Abdominal aortic aneurysm surgery may be associated with renal arterial disruption. Cardiac surgery may be associated with atheroembolism and sustained periods of reduced arterial pressure as well as systemic inflammation.

Other causes

- Nephrotoxins—May cause renal failure via direct tubular injury, interstitial nephritis, or renal tubular obstruction. In patients with AKI, all nephrotoxins that can be stopped should be.
- Rhabdomyolysis—Suggested by myoglobinuria and raised creatine kinase in patients who have suffered crush injury, limb ischemia, coma, or prolonged seizures.
- Glomerular disease—Red cell casts, hematuria, proteinuria, and systemic features (e.g., hypertension, purpura, arthralgia, vasculitis) are all suggestive of glomerular disease. Renal biopsy or specific blood tests (e.g., Goodpasture's syndrome, vasculitis) are required to confirm diagnosis and guide appropriate treatment.
- Hemolytic uremic syndrome—Suggested by hemolysis, uremia, thrombocytopenia and neurological abnormalities.
- Crystal nephropathy—Suggested by the presence of crystals in the urinary sediment. Microscopic examination of the crystals confirms the diagnosis (e.g., urate, oxalate). Release of purines and urate are responsible for acute renal failure in the tumor lysis syndrome.
- Renovascular disorders—Loss of vascular supply may be diagnosed by renography. Complete loss of arterial supply may occur in abdominal trauma or aortic disease (particularly dissection). More commonly, the arterial supply is partially compromised (e.g., renal artery stenosis), and blood flow is further reduced by hemodynamic instability or locally via drug therapy (e.g., NSAIDs, ACE inhibitors). Renal vein obstruction may be due to thrombosis or external compression (e.g., raised intra-abdominal pressure).
- Abdominal compartment syndrome—Suggested by oliguria, a firm abdomen on physical examine, and increased airway pressures (secondary to upward pressure on the diaphragms). Diagnosis is likely when sustained increased intra-abdominal pressures (bladder pressure measured at end-expiration in the supine position) exceed 25 mmHg. However, abdominal compartment syndrome may occur with intra-abdominal pressures as low as 10 mmHg.

Nephrotoxins

The following are some common nephrotoxins:

Allopurinol	Organic solvents
Aminoglycosides	Paraquat
Amphotericin	Pentamidine
Furosemide	Radiographic contrast
Herbal medicines	Sulphonamides
Heavy metals	Thiazides
NSAIDs	

Acute renal failure—management

Identification and correction of reversible causes of AKI is critical. All cases require careful attention to fluid management and nutritional support.

Urinary tract obstruction

Lower tract obstruction requires the insertion of a catheter (suprapubic if there is urethral disruption) to allow decompression. Ureteric obstruction requires urinary tract decompression by nephrostomy or stent. A massive diuresis is common after decompression, so it is important to ensure adequate circulating volume to prevent secondary AKI.

Hemodynamic management

Fluid-responsive AKI may be reversible in its early stage. Careful fluid management to ensure adequate circulating volume and any necessary inotrope or vasopressor support to ensure renal perfusion will help improve chances for renal recovery. Admission to intensive care and use of hemodynamic monitoring should be considered for all patients with AKI and is mandatory for patients not responding to conservative therapy.

Glomerular disease

Specific therapy in the form of immunosuppressive drugs may be useful after diagnosis has been confirmed.

Interstitial nephritis

Acute interstitial nephritis most often results from drug therapy. However, other causes include autoimmune disease, and infection (e.g., Legionella, leptospirosis, streptococcus, cytomegalovirus). Numerous drugs have been implicated but most common are:

- Antibiotics (penicillins, cephalosporins, sulfa, rifampin, quinilones).
- Diuretics (furosemide, bumetanide, thiazides).
- NSAIDs (including selective Cox-2 inhibitors).
- Allopurinol.
- Cimetidine (rarely other H-2 blockers).
- Proton pump inhibitors (omeprazole, lansoprazole).
- Indinavir.
- 5-aminosalicylates.

Urine sediment usually reveals white cells, red cells, and white cell casts. Eosinophiluria is present in about two-thirds of cases and specificity for interstitial nephritis is only about 80 percent. Other causes of AKI in which eosinophiluria is relatively common are rapidly progressive glomerulonephritis and renal atheroemboli.

Discontinuation of the potential causative agent is a mainstay of therapy.

Abdominal compartment syndrome

Abdominal compartment syndrome is a clinical diagnosis in the setting of increased intra-abdominal pressure—pressures below 10 mmHg generally rule it out, whereas pressures above 25 mmHg make it likely. Baseline blood pressure and abdominal-wall compliance influence the amount of intra-abdominal pressure that can be tolerated. Surgical decompression is the only definitive therapy and should be undertaken before irreversible end-organ damage occurs.

Renal replacement therapy

Continuous renal replacement therapy forms the mainstay of replacement therapy in critically ill patients who often cannot tolerate standard hemodialysis due to hemodynamic instability. Standard intermittent hemodialysis is not generally appropriate for hypotensive patients but some centers modify standard dialysis (primarily by prolonging it for many hours) and this may be a reasonable alternative in settings where continuous renal replacement therapy cannot be accomplished. Peritoneal dialysis is not usually is sufficient. Mortality in the setting of acute renal failure in the critically ill is high (50–60 percent). Renal recovery in survivors may be as high as 90 percent but recent studies suggest that sustained renal failure or incomplete renal recovery is more common than previously thought (as many as 50 percent of survivors do not return to baseline renal function following an episode of acute renal failure).

Until recently it was assumed that patients with AKI died not because of AKI itself but secondary to their underlying disease. Several studies, however, have documented a substantial mortality attributable to AKI after controlling for other variables, including chronic illness and underlying severity of acute illness. Table 1.1 lists some of the more important clinical consequences of AKI.

Table 1.1 Clinical consequences of AKI

System	Mechanisms	Complications
Electrolyte disturbances	Hyponatremia Hyperkalemia	CNS (see below) Malignant arrhythmias
Acid-base (Decreased chloride excretion, accumulation of organic anions like PO4, decreased albumin → decreased buffering)	1. Down regulation of Beta receptors, increased iNOS 2. Hyperchloremia 3. Impairing the insulin resistance 4. Innate immunity	1. Decreased cardiac output, blood pressure 2. Lung, intestinal injury, decreases gut barrier function 3. Hyperglycemia. increased protein break down
Cardiovascular	Volume overload	Congestive heart failure Secondary hypertension
Pulmonary	1. Volume overload, decreased oncotic pressure 2. Infiltration and activation of lung neutrophils by cytokines. 3. Uremia	1. Pulmonary edema, pleural effusions 2. Acute lung injury 3. Pulmonary hemorrhage
Gastrointestinal	1. Volume overload 2. Gut ischemia and reperfusion injury	1. Abdominal compartment syndrome 2. Acute gastric and duodenal ulcer → bleeding; impaired nutrient absorption
Immune	1. Tissue edema 2. Decreased clearance of oxygen free radicals 3. White cell dysfunction	Increased risk of infection, delayed wound healing
Hematological	1. Decreased synthesis of RBC, increased destruction of RBC, blood loss 2. Decreased production of erythropoietin, von Willebrand's factor	1. Anemia 2. Bleeding

(continued)

Table 1.1 (continued)

System	Mechanisms	Complications
Nervous system	1. Secondary hepatic failure, malnutrition, altered drug metabolism 2. Hyponatremia, acidosis 3. Uremia	Altered mental status, seizures, impaired consciousness, coma, myopathy, neuropathy → prolonged length on mechanical ventilation
Pharmacokinetics and dynamics	Increased volume of distribution, decreased availability, albumin binding, elimination	Drug toxicity or under dosing

Suggested readings

Bellomo R, Ronco C, Kellum JA, et al.: Acute renal failure—definition, outcome measures, animal models, fluid therapy and information technology needs: the Second International Consensus Conference of the Acute Dialysis Quality Initiative (ADQI) Group. *Crit Care* 2004;8:R204–R212.

Kellum JA: Acute kidney injury. *Crit Care Med* 2008;36:S141–S145.

Uchino S, Kellum JA, Bellomo R, et al.: Acute renal failure in critically ill patients: a multinational, multicenter study. *JAMA* 2005;294:813–818.

Chapter 2

Acute kidney injury in special circumstances

Shamik Shah and Jorge Cerdá

In contemporary practice, most common forms of acute kidney injury (AKI) are associated with sepsis, or occur and after cardiac surgery or radio-contrast administration. Little has changed in the incidence and associated morbidity and mortality over the past four decades. This reflects a lack of effective prevention strategies. Even in survivors, the associated morbidity is associated with escalating health-care utilization and poor long-term outcome. Less commonly, AKI will occur as a result of drug-induced interstitial nephritis. Rarely, AKI will be the initial clinical manifestation of glomerular nephritis in a critically ill patient. After discussing the more common "special circumstances," we will discuss these less common etiologies.

Cardiac surgery and acute kidney injury

Introduction

Acute kidney injury is a known complication of cardiac surgery. However, because of a lack of standardized definition of AKI, the reported incidence in the literature is between 2 percent and 25 percent. Although most patients undergoing cardiac surgery do not need dialysis, studies have shown that even small rises in serum creatinine are associated with increased mortality. Also, despite advances in the understanding, diagnosis and management of this problem, mortality remains very high, between 40 percent and 60 percent.

Pathogenesis

Cardiac surgery may contribute to the development of AKI by several mechanisms:

1. Cellular ischemia:
   a. Blood pressure fluctuations: Mean arterial BP during surgery is often below the limits of autoregulation. Patients undergoing cardiac surgery might also have other co-morbid conditions in which autoregulation is impaired. For example, advanced age, atherosclerosis, ingestion of NSAIDs or ACE inhibitors.

b. Inflammation: Ischemia-reperfusion injury, contact of blood components with cardiopulmonary bypass (CPB) membrane and surgical trauma may all contribute to kidney injury by inciting a systemic inflammatory response.

c. Generation of free radicals: During cardiopulmonary bypass, hemolysis causes the generation of free hemoglobin and iron, which may harm the kidneys.

2. Blood transfusions: Stored RBCs may impair tissue oxygenation, worsen oxidative stress, activate leucocytes, and incite a pro-inflammatory state.

3. Anemia.

Diagnostic criteria

Acute kidney injury is defined according to modified RIFLE (Risk, Injury Failure, Loss, and End stage) or AKIN criteria. See chapter 1.

Biomarkers

Although RIFLE and AKIN classification systems have helped standardize the definition of AKI, they rely on serum creatinine and urine output criteria, which may delay the diagnosis by days. Hence, the search is on for reliable biomarkers that will help in early detection and prognostication of AKI.

Several biomarkers have been evaluated in AKI. See Table 2.1.

Risk factors

Renoprotective interventions

Very few tools are available to the clinician to prevent or treat established AKI. The interventions available can be broadly classified into procedural and pharmacologic. We briefly discuss these interventions:

Table 2.1						
Name	Sample source	Cardiopulmonary bypass (CPB)	Contrast adminis-tration	Critical Care Setting	Kidney Trans-plant (Tx)	Commer-cial Assay
NGAL	Urine	<2 h post CPB	2 h post contrast	48 h pre AKI	12–24 h post Tx	ELISA, ARCHI-TECT
IL-18	Urine	6 h post CPB	Not increased	48 h pre AKI	12–24 h post Tx	ELISA
KIM-1	Urine	12 h post CPB	Not tested	Not tested	Not tested	ELISA
L-FABP	Urine	4 h post CPB	24 h post contrast	Not tested	Not tested	ELISA
NGAL	Plasma	<2 h post CPB	2 h post contrast	48 h pre AKI	Not tested	ELISA, Triage

Procedural interventions

1. *On-pump versus off-pump*: There seems to be little renal benefit of operating patients off-pump.
2. *Hybrid procedures and endovascular stent placements*: These techniques seem to be attractive in theory as they provide the option of avoiding open surgery and cardiopulmonary bypass. For mitral and aortic valve surgeries, retrospective studies show that catheter-based approach and small incisions help reduce the incidence of AKI.
3. *Aprotinin*: It is an antifibrinolytic frequently used in cardiac surgery as a blood-sparing agent. Several studies raised concerns over the safety of this agent in clinical use. Subsequently, it was withdrawn from the market.

Other measures

1. *N-Acetylcysteine (NAC)*: Meta-analyses and RCTs demonstrated that the prophylactic administration of NAC did not reduce the incidence of AKI, postoperative complications, postoperative interventions, mortality, or length of ICU stay.
2. *Vasodilators*: Several trials have looked at the effects of vasodilators in preventing AKI after cardiac surgery. Dopamine, Fenoldopam, Dopexamine, Diltiazem, Prostacyclin, ACE inhibitors, and Mannitol have all been tried but found to be ineffective
3. *Tight glucose control*: Recent single-center studies demonstrated benefit from perioperative tight glucose control, but subsequent studies and meta-analysis involving 3,658 critically ill patients found no mortality benefit or reduction in dialysis rates.
4. *Anemia and hematocrit*: When acute anemia exceeds a threshold of 50 percent reduction from baseline, it is associated with a steadily increasing incidence of adverse outcomes.

Conclusions

Acute kidney injury in cardiac surgery patients is common and is associated with significant morbidity and mortality. Adoption of new definitions will help standardize the diagnosis. Biomarker panels may help in early diagnosis. Although pharmacologic interventions have been largely nonproductive, some procedural changes in surgical techniques may improve outcomes.

Radiocontrast and acute kidney injury

Introduction

Radiocontrast induced acute kidney injury (CIAKI) is one of the commonest causes of iatrogenic renal insufficiency. Although the pathophysiology, risk factors, and natural course are well known, it still causes significant morbidity, mortality, and financial burden.

Pathophysiology

Reduction in renal perfusion involving both tubular and vascular events.

1. Tubular:
   - Marked diuresis and natriuresis stimulating a tubuloglomerular feedback response (TGF). This, in turn, raises renal vascular resistance (RVR) and a decrease in glomerular filtration rate (GFR).
   - Rise in intratubular pressure and blockade of tubules by Tamm-Horsfall proteins.
2. Vascular
   - Stimulae the release of endothelin (ET), vasopressin, angiotensin II, dopamine-1, all potent vasoconstrictors
   - Reduce the activity of renal vasodilators like nitric oxide and prostaglandins.
   - Cause erythrocyte aggregation, resulting in increased blood viscosity and reduced oxygen delivery.
3. Structural changes
   - Vacuolization of proximal tubular cells.
   - Necrosis of the cells of the thick ascending loops of Henle.

Risk factors

- Chronic kidney disease
- Diabetes mellitus.
- Volume depletion
- Nephrotoxic drugs.
- Hemodynamic instability.
- Advanced age.
- Peripheral vascular disease.

Prevention strategies

Choice of contrast medium

Iodinated contrast media can be classified into three groups, based on their osmolarity:

- High osmolar contrast media (HOCM): 2000 mOsm/kg.
- Low osmolar contrast media (LOCM): 600–800 mOsm/kg.
- Iso osmolar contrast media (IOCM): 290 mOsm/kg.

There seems to be an agreement that LOCM are less harmful than HOCM. The evidence is less clear when comparing LOCM and IOCM.

Volume of contrast

It is well known that the volume of contrast used is an important independent factor in the development of CIAKI. Even small volumes can have deleterious effects in patients at high risk.

Intra-arterial versus intravenous administration

Studies have shown that the risk of CIAKI may be higher following intra-arterial when compared to intravenous injection.

Volume expansion

Several studies have compared regimens containing isotonic saline, hypotonic saline, or oral water as bolus or continuous infusion. There is almost unanimous agreement that proper volume management reduces CIAKI. Any regimen that utilizes isotonic saline to increase the ECV by 500 to 1000 ml seems to be effective. However, appropriate caution needs to be observed for patients with congestive heart failure (CHF) or chronic kidney disease (CKD).

Some of the volume-expansion protocols that have been reported in literature are:

1. 0.45 percent saline at 0.5 ml/kg/hr 12 hours preprocedure.
2. Sodium bicarbonate 3 ml/kg/hr 1 hour preprocedure and 1 ml/kg/hr 6 hours postprocedure.
3. 0.9 percent saline. There is consensus that isotonic fluid expansion with 0.9 percent saline is adequate. The benefit of sodium bicarbonate is controversial. Hypotonic solutions such as 0.45 percent saline may be harmful.

N-Acetylcysteine (NAC)

N-acetylcysteine (NAC), a potent antioxidant that scavenges a wide variety of oxygen-derived free radicals, may be capable of preventing CIAKI, both by improving renal hemodynamics and by diminishing direct oxidative tissue damage. However, large studies do not demonstrate benefit.

Sodium bicarbonate

It is believed that pH generation of reactive oxygen species is reduced by alkalization of urine. This can be achieved by the use of sodium bicarbonate. Thus, it is an attractive option for patients undergoing an emergency procedure when there is not enough time to prehydrate with isotonic saline. However, it remains to be proven that $NaHCO_3$ infusion is a good substitute to standard prehydration with isotonic saline, especially in volume-depleted patients.

Dialysis and hemofiltration

Although it is well known that contrast medium is removed by dialysis, there is no good evidence that dialysis can prevent CIAKI. We do not recommend its use.

Gadolinium (Gd)

The risk of CIAKI with iodinated contrast media stimulated the use of magnetic resonance imaging (MRI) with Gadolinium. Free gadolinium is toxic to the liver cells. Hence, several chelates were developed, which ensured that no free gadolinium circulated in blood.

Initial studies suggested that MRI with Gd is relatively safe. The first published report of a nephrogenic fibrosing dermopathy (NFD) in 2000 described thickened skin lesions in patients undergoing dialysis. The causality to Gd was first suggested six years later. Since then, barring macrocyclic chelates, there have been numerous case reports with almost all chelates of Gd, most notably with linear chelates. The half-life of Gd is prolonged in patients with kidney failure. It is also likely that the effect on kidneys is dose dependent. The exact mechanism is not known, but it is believed to be a change in fibroblast activity with Gd.

From the present evidence, it appears that linear compounds should not be used in patients with GFR < 30 ml/min. The use of cyclic compounds appears to be safe, but should be used after weighing the potential risks and benefits.

Acute tubulointerstitial nephritis (TIN)

In patients undergoing kidney biopsy for AKI (a very select group to begin with), 15–27 percent are found to have ATIN.

Etiology
1. Drug Hypersensitivity
   a. Antibiotics:
      i. Beta Lactams—Methicillin, Penicillin, Ampicillin, Oxacillin, Nafcillin.
      ii. Other antibiotics—Sulfonamides, Rifampin, Ethambutol, Polymyxin, Vancomycin, Acylovir, Indinavir, Alpha-Interferon.
   b. NSAIDs—Ibuprofen, Indomethacin, Diclofenac.
   c. Diuretics—Thiazides, Furosemide, Triamterene.
   d. Others—Aspirin, Allopurinol, Carbamezapine, Dipheynlhydantoin, Phenobarbitol, Azathioprine.
2. Infection
   a. Bacterial—Streptococci, Staphylococci, Diphtheria, Brucella, Legionella.
   b. Viral—HIV, Cytomegalovirus, Epstein-Barr virus.
   c. Others—Toxoplasma, Mycoplasma, Rickettsia, Leptospirosis.
3. Immune mediated diseases.
4. Glomerular disease.
5. Idiopathic.

Clinical presentation
1. Abrupt onset of kidney dysfunction, renal insufficiency, and proteinuria—typically in a hospitalized patient with infection, receiving multiple drugs. In such patients, the etiology of AKI is not always clear.
2. The classical triad of fever, rash, and eosinophilia is present in less than 10 percent of patients.
3. Heterogenous.

Lab diagnosis
1. Urinalysis—Presence of leucocytes, leucocyte casts, free RBCs, proteinuria (generally less than 1 g/day), eosinophiluria demonstrated by Wright, Hansel or Giemsa stains.

2. Rapidly rising BUN and Serum Creatinine.
3. Electrolyte imbalances.
4. Normal to enlarged kidney size with increased cortical echogenecity.

Histopathology

Histopathology is the gold standard for diagnosis.
1. Diffuse or patchy inflammatory cell infiltrate within the interstitium comprised of T lymphocytes, monocytes, plasma cells, and eosinophils.

Treatment

1. Removal of offending agent.
2. Conclusive evidence to support the use of immunosuppressive agents as adjunctive therapy is lacking. The following agents have been used with varying success:
   a. Corticsteroids, usually started at a dose of 1 mg/kg and tapered over a period of 1 month.
   b. Cyclophosphamide 1–2 mg/kg/day.
   c. Plasmapheresis—3–4 L exchanges per day for 5 days, and then on alternate days for another week.

Acute glomerulonephritis

Major causes are summarized in the Table 2.2.

Clinical presentation

1. Edema—65 percent.
2. Hypertension—60–80 percent.
3. Decreased urine output—50 percent.
4. Gross Hematuria—30 percent.
5. Nephrotic Syndrome—5 percent.
6. Back pain—5 percent.

Lab diagnosis

1. Urinalysis—Proteinuria, hematuria, casts—100 percent.
2. Serum creatinine > 2 mg/dl—25 percent.
3. Low levels of C3, C4, and/or CH50—See Table 2.2.
4. Nephrotic range proteinuria—10 percent.

Natural history and prognosis

In general, the overall prognosis is very good, as less than 0.5 percent die of the initial disease, and fewer than 2 percent of patients die or develop end-stage renal disease. Both the natural history of the underlying disease and management of its complications contribute to patient outcome. Children have a better prognosis than adults, and patients older than 40 years with rapidly progressive renal failure and crescentic glomerulonephritis have a worse prognosis.

Table 2.2

Low Serum Complement Level	Normal Serum Complement Level
Systemic Diseases	**Systemic Diseases**
Systemic Lupus Erythematosus Cryoglobulinemia Subacute bacterial endocarditis Shunt nephritis	Polyarteritis nodosa Wegener's granulomatosis Hypersensitivity vasculitis Henoch-Schonlein purpura Goodpasture's syndrome Visceral abscess
Renal Diseases	**Renal Diseases**
Acute Poststreptococcal Glomerulonephritis Membranoproliferative Glomerulonephritis • Type I • Type II	IgG-IgA Nephropathy Idiopathic RPGN Anti-GBM disease Pauci-immune

Treatment

The therapy for patients with acute poststreptococcal glomerulonephritis is symptomatic and dependent on the clinical severity of the illness. The major aims of therapy of acute nephritis are control of blood pressure and treatment of volume overload. During the acute phase of the disease, salt and water should be restricted. If significant edema and/or hypertension develop, diuretics should be administered. Furosemide usually provides a prompt diuresis, with reduction of blood pressure. For hypertension uncontrolled by diuretics, vasodilators (i.e., calcium channel blockers or angiotensin converting enzyme [ACE] inhibitors) are usually effective. Steroids or immunosuppressive agents are generally not indicated.

In acute glomerulonephritis secondary to systemic disease, high-dose steroids, diverse immunosuppressive regimens and plasmapheresis are generally indicated.

Hemolytic-uremic syndrome (HUS)

Introduction

It is a devastating, life-threatening clinical syndrome characterized by hemolytic anemia, thrombocytopenia, and progressive renal failure. It is the most common cause of acute kidney injury in children across the world.

Classification

1. **Shiga-like toxin (Stx)–associated HUS (Stx-HUS)**: A disease of children younger than 2–3 years, associated with a food borne infection with verotoxin-producing *Escherichia coli*, especially in summer.

Approximately 75 percent patients present with diarrhea. Hence, this form is denoted as D+ HUS. The other 25 percent do not present with diarrhea and are described as having D-HUS. Acute kidney injury occurs in approximately 70 percent of patients, but 70–85 percent recover renal function.

2. **Non–Stx-associated HUS (non–Stx-HUS)**: Also known as atypical HUS (aHUS) is associated with a number of conditions like genetic factor H deficiency, malignancy, HIV, drugs, and pregnancy. This form of the disease is associated with high mortality rates, permanent renal impairment, and risk of recurrence.

Pathogenesis

In North America and Western Europe, 70 percent of cases of Stx-associated HUS are secondary to *Escherichia coli* serotype O157:H7. Other *E. Coli* serotypes have also been identified. In Asia and Africa, it is associated with Stx-producing *Shigella dysenteriae*.

After oral ingestion of contaminated food or water, *E.Coli* reaches the gut, closely binds to the gut mucosa, and causes cell death. This results in bloody diarrhea. Subsequently, the toxin reaches the systemic circulation and causes microvascular damage at the target organs by blocking protein synthesis and destroying endothelial cells.

Clinical presentation

History

- Abdominal cramps and bloody diarrhea.
- Anuria (55 percent).
- Vomiting (30 to 60 percent).
- Fever (30 percent).
- Irritability, lethargy, convulsions.

Physical findings

- Edema, fluid overload (69 percent).
- Hypertension (47 percent).
- Severe pallor.

Diagnosis

Laboratory Studies

1. Urinalysis: Proteinuria, RBCs and occasionally RBC casts are present.
2. Stool: Presence of *E. Coli* or *Shigella*.
3. Hemoglobin: Severe anemia and presence of schistocytes.
4. Platelet count: Severe thrombocytopenia.
5. Hemolytic work up: Elevated lactate dehydrogenase (LDH), reduced haptoglobin, elevated bilirubin.
6. Kidney function: Elevated BUN, creatinine.

Histologic findings

Occlusive lesions of the arterioles and small arteries and tissue microinfarctions.

Poor prognostic indicators

- Age < 2 years.
- Severe GI prodrome.
- Leucocytosis.
- Early anuria.
- Cortical necrosis.
- Involvement of > 50 percent glomeruli.

Treatment

Supportive therapy

1. Maintain fluid and electrolyte balance.
2. Adequate blood pressure control.
3. Blood transfusions for symptomatic anemia.
4. Bowel rest for hemorrhagic colitis.
5. Prophylactic phenytoin for seizure control in patients with neurologic symptoms.
6. Dialysis: Hemodialysis or peritoneal dialysis as indicated for azotemia.

Antibiotics are not indicated unless bacteremia is present. In S. *Dysenteriae* infection, though, antibiotics must be started early in the course of the disease.

Plasma Exchange or infusion are recommended only for adults with renal and neurologic involvement in the context of Thrombotic Thrombocytopenic Purpura.

Steroids, heparin and antithrombotic agents should be avoided. Bilateral nephrectomy may be helpful in patients with refractory hypertension, major neurologic dysfunction, and persistent thrombocytopenia.

Goodpasture syndrome (anti-GBM disease)

Introduction

It is a rare syndrome of rapidly developing renal failure and pulmonary hemorrhage caused by autoimmunity to a specific component of the glomerular basement membrane (GBM). The reported incidence in Caucasian population is 0.5–0.9 per million per year. Blacks and Asians are affected less than Caucasians.

Pathogenesis

Anti-GBM autoantibodies that are present in the circulation of patients react with the pulmonary (alveolar) and renal (glomerular) basement membranes.

Clinical presentation

History

- Cough.
- Hemoptysis.
- Fatigue.
- Exertional dyspnea.
- Gross hematuria.

Physical findings

- Pallor (due to anemia).
- Edema (fluid overload).
- Dry inspiratory crackles and rhonchi (pulmonary hemorrhage).
- Signs of lung consolidation.
- Heart murmur (due to anemia).
- Hepatomegaly.

Precipitating factors

- Cigarette smoking.
- Respiratory infections.
- Fluid overload.
- Membranous nephropathy.
- Small-vessel vasculitis affecting glomeruli.

Diagnosis

Laboratory studies

1. Urinalysis: Proteinuria, RBCs and occasionally RBC casts are present.
2. Hemoglobin: Severe anemia.
3. WBC count: Leucocytosis.
4. Kidney function: Elevated BUN, creatinine.
5. Anti-GBM titers: Elevated in more than 90 percent patients.
6. Antineutrophilic cytoplasmic antibody (ANCA) titers: raised in about 30 percent of patients. Usually p-ANCA are elevated.

Radiology

Chest radiographs may depict patchy or diffuse infiltrates with sparing of the upper lung fields. These findings may resolve within a few days.

Histology

Lung: Nonspecific findings of hemorrhage with variable degrees of inflammation and fibrosis. Samples obtained during lung biopsy may show IgG staining of the alveolar septum, which is diagnostic for anti-GBM disease.

Kidney: Diffuse glomerulonephritis with focal or complete necrosis of the glomerular tuft and segmental or circumferential cellular crescents surrounding some or all glomeruli. Linear IgG along the GBM can be observed with immunofluorescence testing. Linear C3 along the GBM is present in two-thirds of biopsy samples.

Treatment

A. Removal of Circulating Antibodies.

Plasma exchange: Daily exchange of 1 volume of plasma for 5 percent human albumin for 14 days or until the circulating antibody is suppressed.

B. Prevention of new antibody formation.

Immunosuppressants

i.   **Oral corticosteroids:** Prednisolone is started at 1 mg/kg/24 h orally. The dose is reduced at weekly intervals to achieve one-sixth of the dose by 8 weeks. This dose is then maintained for 3 months, and then tapered and stopped over a period of one month.

ii. **Cyclophosphamide:** For patients younger than 55 years, dose is started at 3 mg/kg/day orally and rounded to the nearest 50 mg. For patients, older than 55 years, the recommended dose is 2.5 mg/kg/day.

iii. **Rituximab:** For patients who are refractory to therapy with plasma exchange and oral steroids and cyclophosphamide, 6 weekly prescribed doses of rituximab at 375 mg/m^2/dose have been recommended.

Suggested readings

Chertow GM, Burdick E, Honour M, et al. Acute kidney injury, mortality, length of stay, and costs in hospitalized patients. *J Am Soc Nephrol.* 2005 Nov;16(11):3365–3370.

McCullough PA, Stacul F, Becker CR, et al. Contrast-Induced Nephropathy (CIN) Consensus Working Panel: executive summary. *Rev Cardiovasc Med.* 2006 Fall;7(4):177–197.

Parikh CR, Devarajan P. New biomarkers of acute kidney injury. *Crit Care Med.* 2008 Apr;36(4 Suppl):S159–S165.

Penfield JG, Reilly RF, Jr. What nephrologists need to know about gadolinium. *Nat Clin Pract Nephrol.* 2007 Dec;3(12):654–668.

Chapter 3

AKI and sepsis

Jorge Cerdá

Sepsis is a highly prevalent complication among critically ill patients, affecting 30–40 percent of the population. Up to 25 percent of those patients have sepsis at ICU admission. Commonest sepsis sources are respiratory and intrabdominal. As the incidence of sepsis increases, so does patient mortality.

Acute kidney injury (AKI) is a frequent complication of sepsis: up to 65 percent of patients with septic shock develop AKI and their mortality is as high as 20–60 percent. The complication is commoner and deadlier when there is delay between the onset of sepsis and septic shock, and initiation of antibiotics. Mortality increases related to septic AKI can extend as far as one year after the insult, even in apparently mild forms of the condition such as community-acquired pneumonia.

The pathogenetic mechanisms of septic AKI are incompletely understood and include a multi-injury pathway of ischemia-reperfusion injury, direct inflammatory injury, coagulation and endothelial cell dysfunction, and apoptosis.

Newer biomarkers may detect renal injury earlier than serum creatinine, especially given that sepsis is associated with decreased creatinine synthesis. Although generally assumed to be associated with tubular necrosis, recent studies have raised questions about the actual nature of renal parenchymal injury in septic AKI.

The intrarenal hemodynamics in septic shock has also been called into question by recent studies demonstrating increased, rather than decreased, renal blood flow (RBF). It is still unclear how RBF distributes within the kidney in this situation, because some vulnerable portions of the tubule may be more severely ischemic such as the thick ascending loop of Henle. Arteriolar pre- and postglomerular dilatation could explain the increased RBF, whereas efferent arteriolar dilatation decreases glomerular capillary filtration pressure and glomerular filtration rate.

Volume resuscitation

Timing and magnitude of volume resuscitation are critical to improve the survival of septic shock patients. The timing of vasopressor and fluid therapy, rather than the specific agent, is decisive to improve outcomes. Once septic shock is recognized, immediate antimicrobial therapy and other measures improve outcomes and avoid complications such as AKI. Such protocols have become the basis for the Surviving Sepsis Campaign and constitute the backbone of contemporary management of septic shock. Application of this protocol has been shown to be associated with significant improvement in survival in the order of a 5.4 percent drop in mortality over the last two years, and decreased incidence and severity of sepsis-induced AKI.

In the initial Early Goal Directed Therapy (EGDT) study by Rivers et al, optimization of cardiac preload, afterload, and contractility to balance oxygen delivery and demand within the first 6 hours postadmission resulted in significant reduction in mortality from 46.5 percent to 30.5 percent in the control and intervention arms of the study, respectively. Although patients assigned to EGDT received more intravenous volume resuscitation within the first 6 hours, at the end of the 72 hours observation both groups received essentially the same volume (13.4 liters).

Recent reevaluation of the EGDT strategy have raised concerns. Three multicentric prospective RCT are currently enrolling patients to answer those questions. From a kidney perspective, concerns include the unreported prevalence of pre-existing renal dysfunction and how many patients eventually required renal replacement therapy (RRT), due to sepsis-induced AKI and/or fluid overload (Figure 3.1).

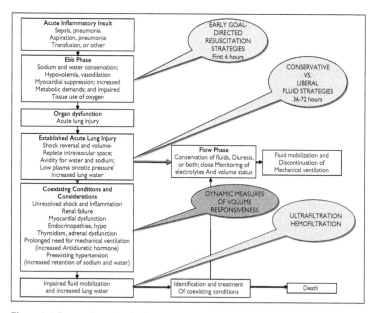

Figure 3.1 Proposed time line for fluid management in AKI.
From Cerda[1]
1. Cerda J, Sheinfeld G, Ronco C. Fluid overload in critically ill patients with acute kidney injury. Blood Purification 2010;29:11–18.

In multiple pediatric and adult studies involving septic patients, fluid overload, oliguria, and late initiation of RRT have been associated with worse patient outcomes. Survival differences are dependent on whether negative fluid balance can be achieved. Similarly, recent studies involving patients with acute respiratory distress syndrome have shown the benefit of a conservative fluid strategy.

Septic patients appear more prone to the development of pulmonary edema and deterioration in pulmonary function. Septic patients developing AKI show initially elevated cardiac-filling pressures, indicating early cardiodepression and a risk of pulmonary edema, illustrating the importance of "cross talk" among injured organs. Given that such patients develop AKI despite fluid expansion, the use of fluid challenges in this patient population may be associated with significant risk. Fluid challenges should be avoided if they do not lead to improvement in renal function or impair oxygenation.

Early application of adequate resuscitation and a subsequent conservative fluid strategy has been shown to be associated with significantly improved patient outcomes.

Optimal management of these patient will, therefore, require initial (within 6 hours) aggressive volume resuscitation, but, as disease progresses, a more conservative fluid strategy is warranted, often requiring diuretics and fluid restriction. As progressive organ failure develops, dynamic estimations of volume status are more accurate than static measurements of central filling pressure, as discussed in chapter 6. If the patient continues to deteriorate and additional organ failures develop, diuretic responsiveness usually ceases, and early institution of RRT usually in the continuous renal replacement therapy (CRRT) becomes necessary to avoid the negative impact of fluid overload.

Vasoconstrictors

Resuscitation strategies include early aggressive fluid expansion and vasopressors, including cathecholamines (norepinephrine, dopamine, epinephrine) and arginine vasopressin (AVP). During AKI, renal autoregulation of RBF is lost and renal perfusion becomes highly dependent on mean perfusion pressure. The subject is extensively reviewed in chapter 7, Pharmacologic Management of AKI, in this volume.

Sepsis management guidelines indicate the early use of the powerful vasoconstrictor norepinephrine (NE) in vasodilatory shock. As mean renal perfusion pressure increases, so does cortical and medullary blood flow, and diuresis.

Concerns with metabolic (i.e., induction of lactatemia) and endocrine (i.e., induction of hyperprolactinemia) effects of epinephrine (EPI) have hampered its use, although recent studies did not demonstrate differences in efficacy. Dopamine at vasoconstrictor doses may be equally powerful as NE, but is associated with higher incidence of arrhythmia than NE. So-called "renal-dose dopamine" offers no benefit and should be abandoned from clinical practice.

During the initial hyperdynamic state, septic shock patients may respond poorly to cathecholamine infusion due to cathecholamine receptor downregulation, inducible nitric oxide synthetase (iNOS) activation and metabolic acidosis. Correction of metabolic acidosis counteracts smooth muscle hyperpolarization induced by acidosis and lactate.

Arginine Vasopressine (AVP), an endogenously released peptide hormone, has emerged as an adjunct to cathecholamines in patients with severe septic shock. Relative deficiency of AVP in sepsis, and its ability to restore cathecholamine receptor responsiveness and counteract iNOS activation and vascular cell hyperpolarization constitute the basis for its use in this context. Addition of AVP to NE allowed for decreased cathecholamine requirements and improved diuresis in small trials, but more recent randomized controlled trials failed to demonstrate a mortality benefit. The common use of AVP as a "cathecholamine-sparing" vasoconstrictor is not supported by evidence. Recent studies have shown that AVP is beneficial in patients with AKI, especially in its early stages ("R" in the RIFLE criteria), possibly supporting its early use in patiens with developing septic AKI.

Recent animal studies with experimental models of sepsis have raised the concern of renal dysfunction and injury induced by AVP.

Cathecholamines and AVP at clinically effective vasoconstrictor doses may induce severe side effects including peripheral and visceral ischemia.

Large placebo-controlled trials of corticosteroids in patients with septic shock have shown conflicting results. Use of low-dose corticosteroids in prolonged infusion is indicated in patients with demonstrated relative endogenous corticosteroid deficiency. It is equally controversial whether corticosteroids improve the effectiveness of AVP.

RRT in sepsis

In sepsis, RRT may be used either as purely renal replacement therapy or as a potential mechanism of immuno-modulation and organ support.

From a renal perspective, methodological questions include timing of initiation, dose of dialysis and RRT modality. Although hypothetically attractive, so far, early initiation of RRT has not been shown benefit. Continuous modalities of RRT (CRRT) do not worsen and often improve hemodynamics in vasodilated septic patients, even when fluid removal is necessary. Control of acidosis often improves vasoconstrictor responsiveness, and lowering of body temperature in the febrile patient contributes to hemodynamic stability. See chapter 10 on Modalities of RRT.

In the last decade, it has been postulated that a high convective dialysis dose improves the management of septic patients. Many water-soluble mediators with anti- and pro-inflammatory action such as TNF alpha, IL-6, IL-8, and IL-10 play an important role in the septic syndrome, and cutting the peaks of soluble mediators through continuous hemofiltration might help restore homeostasis (the "peak concentration hypothesis"). Such benefit has so far not been demonstrated in adequately powered studies, and such techniques are associated with considerable methodological complexity and risk. Other alternatives currently being explored include the use of high-cutoff membranes utilizing plasma filtration coupled with hemadsorption (CPFA) to remove protein-bound solutes and high molecular weight toxins. Hemoperfusion utilizing a filter bound and immobilized Polymyxin B, an antibiotic with high endotoxin affinity was recently shown to be beneficial in a pilot RCT; further larger studies are eagerly awaited.

Finally, ongoing research utilizing "renal tubule cell therapy" (RAD) is currently in Phase II; preliminary results in septic patients have shown promising results and significant decrease in patient mortality.

Selected readings

Vincent JL, Sakr Y, Sprung CL, et al. Sepsis in European intensive care units: results of the SOAP study. *Crit Care Med*. 2006;34:344–353.

Bagshaw SM, Uchino S, Bellomo R, et al. Septic acute kidney injury in critically ill patients: Clinical characteristics and outcomes. *Clin J Am Soc Nephrol*. 2007;2:431–439.

Bellomo R, Wan L, Langenberg C, et al. Septic acute kidney injury: New concepts. *Nephron Exp Nephrol*. 2008;109:e95–e100.

Cerda J, Sheinfeld G, Ronco C. Fluid overload in critically ill patients with acute kidney injury. *Blood Purification*. 2010;29:11–18.

Dellinger RP, Levy MM, Carlet JM, et al. Surviving Sepsis Campaign: International guidelines for management of severe sepsis and septic shock: 2008. *Crit Care Med*. 2008;36:296–327.

Bagshaw SM, Bellomo R, Kellum JA. Oliguria, volume overload, and loop diuretics. *Crit Care Med*. 2008;36:S172–178.

Kellum JA, Cerda J, Kaplan LJ, et al. Fluids for prevention and management of acute kidney injury. *Int J Artif Organs*. 2008;31:96–110.

Bellomo R, Wan L, May C. Vasoactive drugs and acute kidney injury. *Crit Care Med*. 2008;36:S179–S186.

Schrier RW, Wang W. Acute renal failure and sepsis. *N Engl J Med* 2004;351:159–169.

Parrillo JE. Septic shock—vasopressin, norepinephrine, and urgency. *N Engl J Med*. 2008;358:954–956.

Chapter 4

The critically ill patient with chronic kidney disease

Anjali Acharya and Belinda Jim

Background

Chronic kidney disease (CKD) is a common condition affecting about 10 percent of adults over 20 years of age. The incidence of CKD is on the rise. Patients with CKD have a high burden of complex co-morbid conditions, which results in increased hospitalization rates. According to the United States Renal Data System (USRDS), the rates of hospitalization as well as of hospital days per patient-year at risk were 3X higher even among patients with earlier stages of CKD than in the general population.

Definition

The National Kidney Foundation—Kidney Disease Outcomes Quality Initiative (NKF-K/DOQI) workgroup has defined CKD as:

> The presence of markers of kidney damage for ≥ 3 months, as defined by structural or functional abnormalities of the kidney with or without decreased glomerular filtration rate (GFR), that can lead to decreased GFR, manifest by either pathological abnormalities or other markers of kidney damage, including abnormalities in the composition of blood or urine, or abnormalities in imaging tests.

or

> The presence of GFR <60 mL/min/1.73 m^2 for ≥ 3 months, with or without other signs of kidney damage as described above.

Classification of CKD

Table 4.1
• Stage 1 disease is defined by a normal GFR (greater than 90 mL/min per 1.73 m^2) and persistent albuminuria.
• Stage 2 disease is a GFR between 60 to 89 mL/min per 1.73 m^2 and persistent albuminuria.
• Stage 3 disease is a GFR between 30 and 59 mL/min per 1.73 m^2.
• Stage 4 disease is a GFR between 15 and 29 mL/min per 1.73 m^2.
• Stage 5 disease is a GFR of less than 15 mL/min per 1.73 m^2 or end-stage renal disease.

Relationship of CKD and AKI in the ICU

- Acute kidney injury (AKI) occurs in 35–65 percent of ICU admissions. Sepsis accounts for a great percentage of the cases.
- Volume depletion and hypotension are other risk factors for AKI in the ICU.
- Presence of CKD increases the risk of developing AKI. This increase is proportional to stage of CKD, with stages 3–5 showing a much higher rate as compared to those with stages 1–2.

Renal outcomes in patients with CKD

- It is important to remember that the serum creatinine obtained on admission may not reflect the true baseline.
- Renal outcomes as well as patient outcomes have been shown to vary based on baseline serum creatinine on admission to the ICU.
- Several studies have shown that underlying CKD markedly increases the risk of AKI and the risk increases in proportion to the stage of CKD.
- Recent data suggest that AKI contributes to CKD progression.
- Patients with prior CKD who develop AKI are likely to have progression of CKD.
- Patients with AKI and prior CKD who survived hospitalization are more likely to remain dialysis dependent.

Patient outcomes in individuals with CKD

- Mortality rates are substantially high for hospitalized patients with AKI.
- Data on mortality rates based on CKD status in patients who develop AKI is inconclusive, with some studies showing lower mortality rates associated with prior CKD. This was most evident in the lowest tertile of severity of illness in one study.

Specific syndromes in the critically ill ICU patient

This section focuses on the common AKI syndromes seen in the ICU. The patient with CKD is at a higher risk for developing one of these.

Congestive heart failure (CHF)

- Patients with CHF often have CKD, the term cardio-renal syndrome (CRS) is used for this subset of patients.
- Although diuretics remain the mainstay of therapy in acute decompensated heart failure (ADHF), coexisting CKD makes management difficult due to resistance to diuretics. Use of high-dose diuretics is often required, which can lead to AKI and worsening of CKD.
- Although ultrafiltration is frequently used for ADHF, especially when diuretic resistance is encountered, the current consensus is that there is no advantage to ultrafiltration over diuretic use in ADHF.
- Fluid removal may improve renal function and/or restore diuretic responsiveness.

AKI after cardiac surgery

- AKI and worsening of CKD are common after cardiac surgery.
- Preoperative serum creatinine is a major risk factor for AKI after cardiac surgery and allows for identification of high-risk patients.
- There is suggestion that "off pump" cardio pulmonary bypass graft (CABG) reduces development of AKI, though this is yet to be proven in a randomized control trial.
- There is no data to support use of agents such as N-acetyl cysteine (NAC) or mannitol for AKI prophylaxis in patients with CKD at this time.

Contrast-induced nephropathy (CIN)

- CIN is a common complication in the ICU due to frequent diagnostic and therapeutic procedures that use iodinated contrast media.
- CKD, diabetes mellitus, volume depletion and older age are main risk factors.
- Most effective preventive strategies include:

  1. Avoidance of or withholding diuretics, nonsteroidal anti-inflammatory drugs (NSAIDs), angiotensin converting enzyme inhibitors and angiotensin receptor blockers.
  2. Preprocedure volume administration with isotonic crystalloid.
  3. Use of low or iso-osmolality contrast media.

- There is lack of convincing data on the prophylactic use of hemofiltration and hemodialysis to remove contrast material from the circulation in the patient with normal renal function or mild disease and is not recommended in stages 3 and 4 of CKD.

Special considerations in the management of a critically ill patient with CKD

Cardiac troponins in renal disease

The meaning of cardiac troponin enzymes is confusing in the CKD patient. Normally, cardiac troponin I and T (cTnI and cTnT) are elevated in patients with myocardial damage. Though they are the preferred biomarkers for the diagnosis of myocardial injury in patients with normal renal function, their diagnostic utility is unclear in the CKD population. Mild to moderate elevation of serum troponins is common in CKD even in the absence of clinical acute myocardial damage. The exact mechanisms are unknown, but they may include subclinical myocardial damage, leakage of cardiac troponins from myocardial cells into the circulation, left ventricular hypertrophy, and impaired renal clearance of troponin fragments. Interestingly, cTnT remains elevated to a higher degree than cTnI in patients with CKD and ESRD (53–71 percent versus 7–17 percent), perhaps due to the lack of expression of cardiac TnI in noncardiac tissue as compared with cTnT. Despite the controversy in their diagnostic utility, there is abundant evidence that elevations in troponin levels in this population predict an increased risk of cardiovascular outcomes and mortality.

In the critical-care setting, we need to interpret these elevations appropriately.

- Cardiac troponins will rise over 6–8 hours in true myocardial necrosis, regardless of their baseline value.
- Obtain serial troponins.
- cTnT remains elevated to a higher degree than cTnI in CKD/end-stage renal disease (ESRD).
- Dynamic change in cardiac troponins of ≥ 20 percent over their baseline used to define acute coronary syndrome.

Nephrotoxins

Avoidance of nephrotoxins is especially important in the CKD population, due to the already decreased renal reserve. It is important to review the patients' outpatient medications in addition to inpatient medications for their nephrotoxic potential. Common medications such as metformin, ACEI/ARB, spirinolactone, and digoxin should all be used with caution. These medications should either be avoided or have their levels followed closely (e.g., digoxin). Typical nephrotoxins in the ICU include: aminoglycosides, vancomycin, NSAIDs, radiocontrast, intravenous immune globulin (IVIG), hydroxyethyl starches.

Aminoglycosides cause damage to the proximal tubule cell where it is reabsorbed.

- Leads to nonoliguric renal failure.
- Neomycin is associated with the most nephrotoxicity, followed by gentamicin, tobramycin, amikacin, and streptomycin being the least nephrotoxic.
- Risk factors include the type of aminoglycoside, high peak serum levels, cumulative dose, duration and frequency of administration, CKD.
- To minimize aminoglycoside nephrotoxicity, once-daily dosing is preferred with monitoring trough levels to minimize nephrotoxicity.

Vancomycin nephrotoxicity is increasingly being recognized, either alone or in combination with aminoglycosides. These following points are important:

- It is excreted unaltered by glomerular filtration.
- Rates of nephrotoxicity range from 6–30 percent.
- Mechanism of injury is not clear.
- Risk factors include: use of concomitant nephrotoxins, trough level >15ug/mL, increased age, and duration of therapy
- Careful monitoring of renal function and trough levels is mandatory, especially in the event of fluctuating renal function to avoid under- or overdosing.

Nonsteroidal anti-inflammatory drugs (NSAIDs), including the selective COX-2 inhibitors, should be avoided in the ICU patient with CKD for the following reasons:

- They inhibit prostaglandin mediated vasodilatation, which helps to preserve renal blood flow and GFR, especially in volume depletion.
- They may also cause acute interstitial nephritis and nephrotic syndrome (minimal change disease or membranous nephropathy).
- Common culprits include ibuprofen (taken at home), and ketorolac (given in hospital).

Role of diuretics in CKD

Loop diuretics are necessary to manage volume overload in the critically ill CKD patient, especially when there is an acute insult that decreases the GFR. A positive response to diursetics portends better outcome, but this is probably more an indication of milder renal disease. The existence of renal failure requires a higher diuretic dose due to decreased renal perfusion and drug delivery to the kidney, as well as reduced proximal secretion of the drug. These following points will need to be kept in mind in using diuretics in renal failure:

- May need to double or triple the dose of the loop diuretic in CKD.
- Use a combination of a loop diuretic with a thiazide diuretic for improved diuresis.
- Intravenous infusion has been shown to be equivalent in efficacy as bolus injections.
- The only diuretic without a sulfa- moiety is ethacrynic acid, appropriate for those with sulfa allergies.

- Monitor closely for electrolyte abnormalities (hypokalemia, metaboloic alkalosis, hyperuricemia, and hyponatremia).
- Monitor closely for signs of hypoperfusion (hypotension and worsening renal function).
- If the patient no longer responds to diuretics or if the serum urea becomes unacceptably high, consider renal replacement therapy.

Role of angiotensin converting enzyme inhibitors and angiotensin receptor blockers

The angiotensin converting enzyme inhibitors (ACEIs) and the angiotensin receptor blockers (ARBs) are a unique class of medications that may benefit the CKD patient in terms of decreasing intraglomerular hypertension and proteinuria.

Use of ACEIs and ARBs are limited in the critically ill patient with CKD because:

- In the setting of an acute component of renal damage, their use is associated with worsening renal function because it relieves the angiotensin II-mediated vasoconstriction on the efferent arteriole of the glomerulus and reduces the GFR.
- May also result in hyperkalemia.
- In AKI with or without CKD, it is best to discontinue this class of medications until renal function stabilizes.
- Consider prophylactically stopping these medications in the critically ill patient, in anticipation of renal ischemia due to hypotension or other nephrotoxins.

Intravenous immune globulin (IVIG) and hydroxyethyl starch

- For intravenous immune globulin (IVIG) and hydroxyethyl starch, the mechanism of injury appears to be osmotic nephrosis.
- Osmotic nephrosis describes proximal tubule cell swelling due to cytoplasmic vacuolization that results from its inability to break down reabsorbed substances.
- IVIG is often used to manage immune-mediated disorders in the ICU; the stabilizing agent in this product is sucrose which is the culprit.
  - Sucrose, when taken up by proximal tubule cells, causes cellular swelling, luminal narrowing, and occlusion.
  - To minimize nephrotoxicity, administer IVIG over a longer duration or use a nonsucrose preparation.
- Hydroxethyl starches, frequently used to expand volume in hemodynamically unstable patients, are also associated with the development of osmotic nephrosis.
  - High molecular weight hydroxyethyl starches and those with a high C2–C6 molar substitution ratio appear to pose the greatest risk. To minimize nephrotoxiciy with these two agents, we recommend the following:

- To minimize nephrotoxicity, avoid the use of hyperoncotic hydroxethyl starches or use a lower osmolality form.

Tips on initial resuscitation

The initial resuscitation of an unstable, hypotensive patient with chronic kidney disease (CKD) is very similar to that of someone with normal renal function. Our goal is to begin resuscitation immediately if a patient is hypotensive or has an elevated serum lactate of greater than 4 mmol/L aiming to achieve a CVP of 8–12mmHg, mean arterial pressure of > 65mmHg, and urine output of greater 0.5mL/kg/hr. Close monitoring of volume status in CKD patient is crucial with a low threshold for switching to inotropic agents for blood pressure support as the patient is prone to developing volume overload. (See earlier for use of hydroxyethyl starch for volume expansion.)

Anemia management

- Recent data do not support use of erythropoiesis-stimulating agents (ESAs) to treat anemia in the critically ill patient to reduce transfusion requirements, though there was improved survival in trauma patients.
- Erythropoiesis stimulating agent use is not recommended in the critically ill patient with CKD unless the use reflects current guidelines for the noncritically ill CKD patient.
- In CKD, transfusion therapy is recommended when the Hgb is <7.0 g/dL, targeting to 7.0–9.0 g/dL in adults with close monitoring of volume status and use of diuretics.

Deep vein thrombosis (DVT) prophylaxis in CKD patients

Caveats to remember in CKD with the use of low-dose unfractionated heparin (UFH) for DVT prophylaxis are as follows:

- It may potentiate bleeding in patients with gastrointestinal angiodysplasias, and hemorrhagic conversions in patients with pericarditis, both of which are not uncommon in CKD patients. Uremic toxins may further these risks.
- May cause hypoaldosteronism resulting in significant hyperkalemia.
- If low molecular weight heparin (LMWH) is used, a reduction in dose is warranted, especially if used concomitantly with aspirin or clopidogrel.
- Frequent and close monitoring for complications is recommended.
- A mechanical prophylactic option, such as compression stockings or an intermittent compression device, may be used if heparin is contraindicated or not tolerated.

Stress ulcer prophylaxis

- Either a H_2-blocker or proton pump inhibitor (PPI) may be used.
- Development of allergic interstitial nephritis (AIN) after PPI use should be kept in mind, which may worsen existing CKD.

Protein intake

- Providing adequate protein intake in acutely ill CKD patients can be challenging. The recommended protein intake along with the catabolic state raise the blood urea nitrogen levels, which may necessitate initiation of RRT.

Sedation and neuromuscular blockade (NMB)

- Knowledge of pharmacokinetics and side effects and toxicities is crucial in patients with CKD.
- Examples include the following: opioid metabolites, which are active, may be cleared slowly in CKD. Prolonged use of propylene glycol as a vehicle to administer propofol can result in development of an anion gap acidosis. This may worsen acidosis from CKD.
- Use of depolarizing NMB agents can cause hyperkalemia, which can pose a problem in patients with CKD.

Glucose control

- If use of insulin is required, it is important to remember that half-life of insulin is prolonged in patients with CKD. In addition, renal gluconeogenesis is impaired. Both these factors predispose CKD patients to hypoglycemia. Therefore, starting with a small dose of insulin is recommended.

Consideration for limitation of support

- Advance care planning with patients and families is crucial in the CKD patient due to the high burden of co-morbidities in such a patient. It is important to discuss likely outcomes and set realistic expectations.
- Initiation of RRT and its implications, as well as a "time-limited" dialysis option should be discussed.

Suggested readings

Charytan C, Kaplan A, Paganini E, et al. Role of the nephrologist in the Intensive Care Unit: *AJKD*. 2001;38(2):426–429.

Corwin HL, Gettinger A, Fabian TC, et al. EPO Critical Care Trials Group: Efficacy and safety of epoetin alfa in critically ill patients. *N Engl J Med*. 2007;357:965–976.

Kanderian AS, Francis GS. Cardiac troponins and chronic kidney disease. *Kidney International*. 2006;69:1112–1114.

Lee PT, Chou KJ, Liu CP, et. al. Renal protection for coronary angiography in advanced renal failure patients by prophylactic hemodialysis: A randomized controlled trial. *J Am Coll Cardiol*. 2007;50:1015–1020.

Navaneethan SD, Singh S, Appasamy S, et al. Sodium bicarbonate therapy for prevention of contrast-induced nephropathy: A systematic review and meta-analysis. *Am J Kidney Dis*. 2009;53:617–627.

U.S. Renal Data System, USRDS 2000 Annual Data Report): Atlas of End-Stage Renal Disease in the United States, National Institutes of Health, National Institute of Diabetes and Digestive and Kidney Diseases, Bethesda, MD, 2000:AD-PMID-11077892

Wang AY-M, Lai K-N. Use of cardiac biomarkers in end-stage renal disease. *J Am Soc Nephrol*. 2008;19:1643–1652.

Wu AH, Jaffe AS, Apple FS, et al. National Academy of Clinical Biochemistry Laboratory Medicine Practice Guidelines: Use of cardiac troponin and B-type natriuretic peptide or N-terminal proB-type natriuretic peptide for etiologies other than acute coronary syndromes and heart failure. *Clin Chem*. 2007;53:2086–2096.

Chapter 5

Principles of fluid management

Rinaldo Bellomo and Sean M. Bagshaw

Introduction

The control and optimization of fluid balance is a clinically important component of continuous renal replacement therapy (CRRT). Inadequate fluid removal is associated with peripheral edema and vital organ edema (i.e. pulmonary edema). Such edema can retard weaning from mechanical ventilation or compromise wound healing. Fluid overload has been identified as an independent predictor of increased mortality in critically ill patients and is clearly undesirable. Similarly, excessive fluid removal may contribute to hypovolemia with increased doses of vasopressor drug therapy, exposing the patients to the risks of unnecessary beta- and alpha-receptor stimulation. Hypovolemia may induce hypotension and, thereby, possibly aggravate organ injury and, specifically, retard or block renal recovery. Accordingly, careful clinical assessment of the patient's fluid status and careful prescription of CRRT to optimize fluid balance, together with frequent review of such assessment and prescription represent a key aspect of best practice in the field of CRRT.

Patient fluid balance: This term refers to the total balance over a 24-hour period of fluids administered (intermittent drugs, continuous infusions of drugs, blood, blood products, nutrient solutions, additional fluids) and measurable fluids removed (drainage from chest or abdomen, urine—if present, blood loss and excess fluid removed by the CRRT machine).

Machine (CRRT) fluid balance: this term refers to the total balance over a 24-hour period of fluids administered by the CRRT machine (dialysate or replacement fluid or both depending on the technique and any additional anticoagulant infusion) and fluids removed by the CRRT machine (spent dialysate or ultrafiltrate or both depending on the technique).

Effluent: the total amount of fluid discarded by the machine. In continuous veno-venous hemofiltration (CVVH), this is the same as ultrafiltrate. In continuous veno-venous hemodialysis (CVVHD), this is equal to the spent dialysate + any additional ultrafiltrate generated by the machine. In continuous venovenous hemodialfiltration (CVVHDF), this is the same as the sum of spent dialysate and ultrafiltrate discarded by the machine (also called spent ultradialfiltrate).

Dry weight: This is the patient's normal/optimal weight before the onset of illness. This weight is often available in detail in elective operative patients when it is typically measured before the operation. In other cases, it might need to be estimated.

Edema: This term refers to the accumulation of excess fluid in the extracellular compartment. In the subcutaneous tissue, it can be detected by the phenomenon of pitting of the skin under pressure. In the lungs, if significant, it can be detected by radiography.

Assessment of fluid status: This term refers to the clinical process of estimating the patient's intravascular and extravascular fluid status. Such assessment is complex and imperfect. It requires consideration of vital signs, invasive and noninvasive hemodynamic measurements, information of fluid balance and body weight, and radiological information. Such assessment is necessary to guide fluid balance prescription during CRRT.

Approach to fluid balance during CRRT

The prescription of CRRT-related fluid management and its integration into overall patient fluid management can be assisted by a specific order chart (Table 5.1) for the machine fluid balance.

Table 5.1 will tell the nurse how to set the machine and how to achieve the planned hourly fluid balance. However, in ICU, the fluid needs of the patients are not static and require frequent review. For example, should the same patient require the administration of 600 ml of fresh frozen plasma over 2 hours prior to an invasive procedure, necessary adjustments to the order should be made with specification for the duration of change and the reasons (Table 5.2).

The fluid balance prescription related to the machine can be usefully related to the patient, and a fluid balance prescription describing the overall patient fluid balance goal for a 12-hour time period is useful for informing the nurse what the broad goals of fluid therapy are in a given patient. This may be expressed in an additional prescription attached to the previous machine fluid balance chart (Table 5.3).

Practical considerations

The preceding goals can be achieved by means of physician and nursing education and by ensuring that no CRRT session can be started unless such orders are clearly and legibly written, signed, and accompanied by the physician's printed

Table 5.1 Prescription of machine fluid balance during CRRT					
Technique	Dialysate flow rate	Replacement fluid flow rate	Effluent flow rate	Anticoagulant infusion flow rate	Machine fluid balance
CVVHDF	1000 ml/hr	1000 ml/hr	2300 ml/hr	100 ml/hr	−200 ml/hr

Table 5.2 Alteration of CRRT fluid balance prescription					
Technique	Dialysate flow rate	Replacement fluid flow rate	Effluent flow rate	Anticoagulant infusion flow rate	Machine fluid balance
CVVHDF	1000 ml/hr	1000 ml/hr	2600 ml/hr	100 ml/hr	−500 ml/hr (for 2 hours only during FFP treatment)

Table 5.3 Patient fluid balance prescription				
Patient	Medical record number	Overall fluid balance from midnight to 12:00 (noon)	Overall fluid balance from 12:00 (noon) to midnight	Right atrial pressure notification range
Name	00123	−1000 ml	−1000 ml/hr	< 6 or > 15 mmHg

name and contact number. They also require the regular recording of fluid balance on an hourly basis and its correct final addition of fluid losses and gains. This can be done in a computerized system or added by the nurse at the bedside using a pocket calculator and then charted. This process allows the creation of a running hourly balance, which is useful in ensuring that progress is being made at the appropriate speed, in the appropriate direction and to the prescribed amount.

Expected outcomes, potential problems, cautions, benefits

The expected outcome of a systematic process for the prescription, delivery, and monitoring of fluids during CRRT is the ability to ensure that the patient will receive prescribed therapy in a safe and effective manner. This approach will minimize errors and their consequences (persistent fluid overload or dangerous intravascular volume depletion).

Despite this careful approach, problems can still arise. A relatively common problem is related to off-time (time during which CRRT is not operative due to filter clotting or an out-of-ICU procedure or investigation). Under such circumstances, the planned fluid removal cannot proceed as planned. If the patient has 5 hours of off-time, then the consequence may be that close to one liter of planned fluid removal fails to occur (assuming fluid balance of −200 ml/hr). Moreover, during this off-time, patients may be administered additional fluid that will counter earlier fluid balance goals. If this happens, the physician and the nurse need to be alert to the consequences and respond appropriately. This may require an adjustment in fluid removal during the ensuing 12 or 24 hours, which safely compensates for the off-time by increasing the hourly fluid removal by, for example, an extra 100 ml/hr. Due consideration needs to be paid to specific patients in whom such fluid removal may be problematic. However, typically, machine fluid removal rates of 300–400 ml/hr are well tolerated in fluid overloaded patients. Nonetheless, caution should be exerted, and the patient's condition should be reviewed frequently.

Another relatively common problem relates to frequent interruptions of therapy due to machine alarms. In some patients who are agitated or who have frequent leg flexion in the presence of a femoral access catheter or who sit up and move in the bed in the presence of a subclavian access device, the machine pressure alarms may be frequently triggered. In addition, other alarms related to substitution fluids bag or waste bag changes interrupt treatment. This may lead to periods of 5–10 minutes over an hour, and over a day these create "lost treatment time" and failure to achieve fluid balance goals. It is often prudent to prescribe a greater fluid loss than desired to compensate for these factors. Most machines allow the operator to check what the actual fluid removal achieved was over a given time period. Such checks should be done to ensure that the correct fluid removal is entered into the fluid balance calculations; many nursing protocols mandate fluid balance check each hour particularly for inexperienced nurses.

The benefits of such continuous monitoring of fluid delivery and removal are many. They include frequent patient assessment, vigilance with regard to other simultaneous therapies, attention to detail, avoidance of dangerous swings in fluid status, and competent and detailed machine operation.

Summary or conclusion

Attention to fluid balance during CRRT is of great clinical importance. Inadequate fluid removal leads to clinical complications, especially in relation to weaning from mechanical ventilation. Excessive fluid removal can cause hypovolemia and hypotension and retard renal recovery. Best practice in this field can only be achieved by a systematic combination of frequent and thoughtful assessment, attention to detail, rigorous and vigilant monitoring of fluid input and output, and clear and explicit description and prescription of the goals of therapy with regard to both machine settings and patient management.

Suggested readings

Bagshaw S, Baldwin I, Fealy N, Bellomo R. Fluid balance error in continuous renal replacement therapy: A technical note. *Int J Artif Organs*. 2007;30:435–440.

Bagshaw S, Bellomo R. Fluid resuscitation and the septic kidney. *Curr Opin Crit Care*. 2006;12:527–530.

Bagshaw SM, Bellomo R. The influence of volume management on outcome. *Curr Opin Crit Care*. 2007;13:541–548.

Bagshaw SM, Brophy PD, Cruz D, et al. Fluid balance as a biomarker: Impact of fluid overload on outcome in critically ill patients with acute kidney injury. *Crit Care*. 2008;12:169.

Chapter 6

Functional hemodynamic monitoring

Xaime García and Michael R. Pinsky

Hemodynamic monitoring is the act of assessing the cardiovascular values, such as blood pressure, heart rate, and cardiac output, and their patterns. Its clinical utility rests in defining variations from normal ranges and the constellation of abnormal patterns that define specific pathological cardiovascular states, such as hypovolemia, heart failure, and sepsis. Functional hemodynamic monitoring, on the other hand, is the assessment of the dynamic interactions of hemodynamic variables in response to a defined perturbation. Such dynamic responses result in emergent parameters of these commonly reported variables that greatly increase the ability of these measures to define cardiovascular state and predict response to therapy.

Potentially, any hemodynamic monitoring measure could have its data applied functionally. The analogy of monitoring to functional monitoring is similar to the relationship of the electrocardiogram (ECG) to the stress ECG. The stress ECG adds ischemic potential to this monitoring tool. At the present time, the primary types of functional hemodynamic monitoring for which clinical trials have shown usefulness are related to identifying occult cardiovascular insufficiency (compensated shock) and predicting volume responsiveness.

The identification of cardiovascular insufficiency comes from inspection of tissue O_2 saturation (StO_2) changes in response to a vascular occlusion test (VOT), whereas identification of volume responsiveness comes from quantifying the impact of positive-pressure ventilation in left ventricular stroke volume variation and arterial pulse pressure variation (SVV and PPV, respectively) or, during spontaneous ventilation, the effect of spontaneous inspiration of central venous pressure changes or the changes in mean cardiac output in response to a passive leg raising (PLR) test.

Identification of cardiovascular insufficiency: Assessing cardiovascular reserve by noting changes in StO₂ to a VOT

Noninvasive measurement of StO_2 using near-infrared spectroscopy has been shown as a valid method to assess the microcirculation status, especially in septic and trauma patients. The absolute StO_2 value has a limited discriminating capacity, because StO_2 remains within the normal range until shock is quite advanced. However, the addition of a dynamic ischemic challenge, such as the VOT, improves and expands the predictive ability of StO_2 to identify tissue hypoperfusion. The VOT measures the effect of total vascular occlusion-induced tissue ischemia and release on downstream StO_2. StO_2 is measured on the thenar eminence and transient rapid vascular occlusion of the arm by sphygmomanometer inflation to 30 mmHg above systolic pressure is performed either for a defined time interval, usually 3 minutes, or until StO_2 declines to some threshold minimal value, usually 40 percent. The deoxygenation rate reflects the local metabolic rate and mitochondrial function, and the rate of reoxygenation rate reflects local cardiovascular reserve and microcirculatory flow.

Volume responsiveness

A primary resuscitation question is whether patients will increase their cardiac output in response to intravascular volume infusion. Volume responsiveness is arbitrarily defined as a ≥15 percent in cardiac output in response to a 500 ml bolus fluid challenge. Although the presence of fluid responsiveness in a subject does not equate for the need to give fluids, it does define that, if fluids are infused, CO will increase. Importantly, all static hemodynamic estimates of preload, including central venous pressure, pulmonary artery occlusion pressure, right ventricular end-diastolic volume, and left ventricular end-diastolic area are not predictive of volume responsiveness. In the assessment of preload responsiveness, one needs to measure functional parameters. The simplest method to assess preload responsiveness is to give a small-volume intravenous bolus and evaluate the hemodynamic response. A patient is considered a volume responder if there is a significant increase in flow-dependent variables like CO, mean arterial pressure, SvO_2, or urine output. The main problem with performing the fluid challenge is that only half of hemodynamically unstable patients will increase CO after the fluid challenge, and in half of those patients who are not fluid responders, the volume charge may be injurious (e.g., cor pulmonale or left ventricular failure). Also the fluid challenge takes time to perform and evaluate.

For this reason, alternative methods to guide volume responsiveness gained interest in the acute-care setting.

Passive leg raising

Passive leg raising (PLR) to 30° for 3 minutes while keeping the head at 0° transiently increases venous return to the heart. In fluid responders, one sees a ≥ 15 percent transient increase of CO. The advantage of the PLR maneuver is that it can be done quickly without special equipment, it is reversible in the intravascular volume shifts that are proportional to body size of each subject, and it can be repeated safely over time. It can be performed in patients breathing spontaneously and also in the absence of sinus rhythm; thus it becomes the universal functional hemodynamic volume challenge. Its primary limitation is that, in profoundly hypovolemic patients, the transfer of blood may be to too small to elicit a CO response, though this is a rare event, even in those in severe hemorrhagic shock.

Changes in left ventricular output during positive-pressure ventilation

During the inspiratory phase of positive-pressure ventilation, intrathoracic pressure increases passively, increasing right atrial pressure, causing venous return to decrease, decreasing right ventricular output, and after two or three heart beats, increasing left ventricular output if both ventricles are volume responsive. Thus, in preload dependent patients, cyclic changes in left ventricular stroke volume and its coupled arterial pulse pressure are seen, and the magnitude of the changes is proportional to volume responsiveness. The associated SVV and PPV are quantified in various ways, depending on whether these are measured by minimally invasive cardiac output monitors (e.g., PiCCO, LiDCO, FloTrac) or by direct examination of the pressure or flow profiles. In general, both are defined as the ratio of the maximal minus the minimal values to the mean values, usually averaged over 3 or more breaths. Numerous studies have documented that an SVV >10 percent or a PPV>13–15 percent on a tidal volume of 8 ml/kg or greater is highly predictive of volume responsiveness. Pulse pressure ventilation is easier to measure than SVV because it only requires inspection of the arterial pressure waveform, whereas to directly measure SVV, Doppler echocardiography is needed or analogue estimates of left ventricular stroke volume from interpellation of the arterial pressure waveform.

Because the pulse oximetry plethysmographic signal is directly influenced by the peripheral arterial pressure waveform, the beat-to-beat changes in the amplitude of the plethysmographic pulse wave (ΔP_{PLET}) are assumed to be the result of the beat-to-beat changes in stroke volume transmitted to the arterial blood flow with a similar fluid responsive threshold of 14 percent. Though an easy and noninvasive method for predicting volume responsiveness, the pleth signal is often lost in circulatory shock, limb tremor, hypothermia, or arterial vasoconstriction.

Furthermore, quantifying only systolic pressure variation (SPV), an earlier proposed method, is also predictive of volume responsiveness though with a lesser predictive power.

Based on the same physiologic concept of the increase in thoracic pressure during positive pressure ventilation, some flow measurements of inferior vena caval or superior vena caval flow variations using Doppler techniques also demonstrate excellent discrimination in predicting volume responsiveness. Here, positive-pressure inspiration associated caval collapse, quantified as a decrease in the caval diameter of > 12 percent, predicts volume responsiveness. The respiratory changes in left ventricular stroke volume are reflected in the peak velocity of aortic flow that can be easily measured beat-to-beat

Table 6.1

IPPV-induced changes in flow

a) Left ventricular output (~>10–15 percent)

 • Pulse pressure variation

 • Stroke volume variation

 • Amplitude of the plethysmographic pulse wave

 • Change in peak velocity of aortic flow (transesophagic echocardiography/USCOM®)

b) Venous collapse (~>10–15 percent)

 • Respiratory variation in inferior vena cava diameter (transthoracic echocardiography)

 • Superior vena cava collapsibility (transesophageal echocardiography)

using transesophageal echocardiography or transcutaneous continuous-wave Doppler (USCOM system), with threshold values ≥ 12 percent in peak velocity (ΔV peak), predicting volume responsiveness.

All the existing and validated means to assess volume responsiveness in patients on positive-pressure ventilation are listed in Table 6.1.

Although powerful diagnostic tools, these parameters are highly dependent on the cyclic changes in intrathoracic pressure being regular and great enough to alter central venous pressure. Thus, tidal volumes of ≤6 ml/kg or the imposition of variable spontaneous inspiratory efforts often result in false negative PPV and SVV values. Similarly, all these techniques assume a fixed heart rate. Thus, in the setting of atrial fibrillation or frequent premature ventricular contractions, these measures become inaccurate. In these settings, one can always perform a PLR maneuver. A potentially interesting use of the PPV and SVV analysis would be to identify when excessive amounts of positive end-expiratory pressure were being applied, because hyperinflation would resemble hypovolemia in terms of increasing PPV or SVV. However, this application has not been validated.

Assessing fluid responsiveness during spontaneous breathing

During spontaneous inspiration, intrathoracic pressure decreases and it allows an increase in venous return. Therefore, if right ventricular function is preserved and transfers this increased blood through the pulmonary circulation, then right atrial pressure will decrease with inspiration. An inspiratory decrease in right atrial pressure of more than 1 mmHg when intrathoracic pressure decreases more than 2 mmHg may predict preload responsiveness in patients with spontaneous breathing. Though measuring such small changes in right atrial pressure are often difficult, greater negative swings in right atrial pressure are usually easier to identify of the pressure waveform. Finally, as listed earlier, if CO is being monitored, the PLR maneuver can also be used in spontaneously breathing patient.

Applicability of functional hemodynamic monitoring

Numerous clinical trials have attempted to document improved patient outcome using hyper-resuscitation techniques guided by measured hemodynamic variables in patients with existing circulatory shock and its associated organ injury. They were uniformly unsuccessful. However, when the same protocols were recently applied in a proactive fashion in high-risk surgery patients with the goal of PPV minimization, Lopes et al. (2007) documented markedly reduced morbidity. Similarly, Pearse et al. conducted a study to evaluate the effect of postoperative goal-directed therapy in postoperative high-risk patients. Targeting an oxygen delivery index > 600 mL/kg/min they were able to reduce both postoperative complications and median duration of hospital stay.

These two examples show that functional hemodynamic monitoring has an important place in the correct management of critically ill patients and its applicability in shock resuscitation.

Suggested readings

Berkenstadt H, Margalit N, Hadani M, et al. Stroke volume variation as a predictor of fluid responsiveness in patients undergoing brain surgery. *Anesth Analg.* 2001;92:984–989.

Cannesson M, Besnard C, Durand PG, et al. Relation between respiratory variations in pulse oximetry plethysmographic waveform amplitude and arterial pulse pressure in ventilated patients. *Critical Care.* 2005;9:R562–R568.

Feissel M, Michard F, Mangin I, et al. Respiratory changes in aortic blood velocity as an indicator of fluid responsiveness in ventilated patients with septic shock. *Chest.* 2001;119:867–873.

Feissel M, Richard F, Faller JP, et al: The respiratory variation in inferior vena cava diameter as a guide to fluid therapy. *Intensive Care Med.* 2004;30:1834–1837.

Gomez H, Torres A, Polanco P, et al. Use a non-invasive NIRS during vascular occlusion test to assess dynamic tissue O_2 saturation response. *Intensive Care Med.* 2008;34:1600–1607.

Michard F, Boussat S, Chemla D, et al. Relation between respiratory changes in arterial pulse pressure and fluid responsiveness in septic patients with acute circulatory failure. *Am J Respir Crit Care Med.* 2000;162:134–138.

Lopes RL, Oliveira MA, Pereira VOS, et al. Goal-directed fluid management based on pulse pressure variation monitoring during high-risk surgery: a pilot randomized controlled trial. *Crit Care.* 2007;11(5):R100.

Magder SA, Georgiadis G, TUC C. Respiratory variations in right atrial pressure predict response to fluid challenge. *J Crit Care.* 1992;7:76–85.

Michard F, Teboul JL. Predicting fluid responsiveness in ICU patients: A critical analysis of the evidence. *Chest.* 2002;121:2000–2008.

Monnet X, Teboul JL. Passive leg raising. *Intensive Care Med.* 2008;34:659–663.

Pearse R, Dawson D, Fawcet J, et al. Early goal-directed therapy after major surgery reduces complications and duration of hospital stay. A randomised, controlled trial. *Crit Care*. 2005;9:R687–R693.

Perel A. Assesisng fluid responsiveness by the systolic pressure variation in mechanically ventilated patients: systolic pressure variation as a guide to fluid therapy in patients with sepsis-induced hypotension. *Anesthesiology*. 1998;89:1309–1310.

Pinsky M R, Payen D. Functional hemodynamic monitoring. *Crit Care*. 2005;9(6):566–572.

Thiel S, Kollef M, Isakow W. Non-invasive stroke measurement and passive leg raising predict volume responsiveness in medical ICU patients: an observational cohort study. *Critical Care*. 2009;13:R111.

Vieillard-Baron A, Chergui K, Rabiller A. Superior vena cava collapsibility as a gauge of volume status in ventilated septic patients. *Intensive Care Med*. 2004;30:1734–1739.

Chapter 7

Pharmacologic therapy in acute kidney injury

Jorge Cerdá

Introduction

The incidence of acute kidney injury (AKI) critically ill patients is high; its diagnosis is difficult and often late. Given the absence of effective therapeutic means to restore renal function, clinicians can only optimize fluid volume and composition, hemodynamic and nutritional support, and apply renal replacement therapy (RRT) whenever indicated, while awaiting spontaneous renal recovery. In this setting, pharmacologic therapy is essential for patient management, timely initiation of RRT and renal functional recovery.

This chapter will successively focus on the pharmacological interventions geared to the prophylaxis and the treatment of established AKI. Chapter 8 will discuss drug dosing and pharmacokinetics in patients with AKI.

Shock and AKI

Several measures have been suggested to minimize the development of AKI in the patient in shock, but none carry a high-grade recommendation. These include prompt resuscitation of the circulation with volume expansion and maintenance of organ perfusion pressure using vasopressors in vasodilatory hypotension. These measures constitute the basis of the Surviving Sepsis Campaign, as discussed in chapter 3.

Volume expansion

Beyond the need to optimize hemodynamics and the prevention of acid base and electrolyte abnormalities, there is little evidence supporting the preferential use of crystalloids, human serum albumin, gelatine-derived colloids, or lower molecular weight hydroxy-ethyl starch (HES) for renal protection. High-volume resuscitation with 0.9 percent saline solution may induce hyperchloremic metabolic acidosis.

It is incompletely understood how volume expansion increases systolic volume and cardiac output; in addition to increasing preload and end-diastolic volume, volume expansion may induce improved contractility and decreased afterload.

Prophylactic volume expansion has been recommended to prevent AKI induced by certain drugs including amphotericin B; antivirals such as foscarnet, cidofobir, and edefovir; certain drugs causing crystal nephropathy such as indinavir, acyclovir, and sulfadiazine; and to decrease the toxicity of certain chemotherapeutic agents such as cisplatinum.

Vasopresors and inotropes

Tables 7.1 and 7.2 summarize the principal pharmacologic effects of commonly used vasopressors and inotropes. Vasopressors should be used to maintain mean arterial pressure (MAP) above 60–65 mmHg, but target MAP should be individualized whenever possible. Given that, during developing or established AKI, the normal autoregulation of renal blood flow is lost, renal perfusion becomes highly dependent on perfusion pressure. Additionally, given the complexity of intrarenal circulation, "renal vasodilation" may not be necessarily beneficial if it is restricted to the cortex and results in additional ischemia of areas in which tissue oxigenation is highly flow-dependent, such as the outer medulla.

The use of vasopressors in patients with or at risk of AKI is fraught with controversy. Although practitioners are commonly fearful of inducing intrarenal vasconstriction and hypoxic injury, experimental and clinical data show the opposite: norepinephrine (NE) infusion in the setting of vasodilatory shock improves renal blood flow and diuresis.

Table 7.1 Primary effects of alpha and beta-adrenergic stimulation	
Beta	Increased force of contraction
	Increased heart rate
	Vasodilation
	Increased hepatosplenic blood flow
	Increased cellular metabolism
Alpha	Vasoconstriction—increase in blood pressure
	Decreased blood flow (increased afterload)
	Decreased heart rate (baroreflex)
	Increased cerebral blood flow
	Decreased renal and hepatosplachnic blood flow
Dopamine 1	Renal and mesenteric vasodilation
Dopamine 2	Norepinephrine release from sympathetic nerve endings
	Inhibition of prolactin release
	Antinausea effects

Table 7.2 Relative effects of common vasoactive medications on adrenergic receptors

Agent (typical dosages)	β-1	β-2	α-1
Isoproterenol (0.01–0.1 µg/kg/min)	+++	+++	O
Norepinephrine (0.05–1 µg/kg/min)	++	0	+++
Epinephrine (0.05–2 µg/kg/min)	+++	++	+++
Phenylephrine (0.5–5 µg/kg/min)	O	O	+++
Dopamine* (1–20 µg/kg/min)	+(++)	+	+(++)
Dobutamine (2.5–20 µg/kg/min)	+++	+	+

Table 7.2 shows dopamine effects at "high dose" typically greater than 3–5 µg/kg/min (shown in parenthesis). 0: no effect; +: minimal effect; ++: moderate effect; +++: substantial effect.

When used at doses necessary to reverse distributive shock, less potent vaso-constrictors such as dopamine are not safer and may actually be associated with greater risks such as arrhythmia and sudden death, especially in patients with cardiogenic shock. Although both NE and dopamine, at equipotent doses can increase blood pressure in shock situations, the use of dopamine has been pur-ported to be associated with special benefits including increased hepato-splachnic and renal blood flow, but evidence of such benefit is lacking. Dopamine has additional undesirable effects including hyperprolactinemia, although the clinical relevance of these effects is questionable. A recently completed randomized control trial comparing NE and dopamine showed no difference in efficacy and a greater number of adverse events with dopamine.

As shown in multiple studies and meta-analyses, the use of "renal dose" dopa-mine (3–5 µg/kg/min) for the prevention or treatment of AKI cannot be justified: its use should be eliminated from routine clinical use.

Norepinephrine (up to 1 µg/kg/min) infusion is routinely used in the the vasodilated patient in shock after volume re-expansion is complete, and it is the recommended first line drug in septic shock. Other vasopressor drugs such as epinephrine and phenylephrine may be similar in efficacy to NE, but experience and available evidence on their use is less abundant. Epinephrine has been as-sociated with metabolic disturbances including hyperglycemia, hyperlactatemia, acidosis and hyperkalemia, but studies are small and fraught with methodo-logical problems. Epinephrine at doses of 0.4 µg/kg/min has been shown to increase cardiac output and MAP, heart rate and myocardial contractility, but may also cause severe peripheral vasocontriction and ischemia in most regional circulations.

Arginine vasopressin (AVP) at low doses (0.01 to 0.04 IU/min) is increasingly popular in the management of NE-refractory shock, but has not been convincingly shown to improve survival, prevent AKI, or ameliorate kidney function. In septic shock, patients may experience a relative deficiency of AVP; this fact and the efficacy of AVP to overcome nitric-oxide induced vasodilation and catecholamine receptor-down regulation has provided the rationale for its use in septic shock. Recently completed randomized trials failed to demonstrate superiority of AVP over NE, but the studies did not address its common clinical use as a NE-sparing vasopressor. Recent studies have shown that AVP compared to NE decreases the progression of AKI to its most severe stages among patients with septic shock. It should be emphasized that, at larger doses, AVP can induce severe peripheral and mesenteric ischemic injury.

Terlipressing (glycine vasopressin, 1 to 2 mg every 6 hours), a longer half-life vasoconstrictor that can be used subcutaneously, has been found effective in patients with AKI associated with severe liver failure (hepatorenal syndrome type 1), but it is unclear whether this drug is superior to NE or AVP in this setting.

In summary, although still controversial, the use of vasoconstrictors in patients with hypotensive vasodilation despite fluid resuscitation appears warranted, because it has been proven safe and effective when applied in individualized fashion. In these patients, restoration of blood pressure to improve organ perfusion should be achieved with prompt use of norepinephrine and sustained until vasodilation resolves. Renal dose dopamine is not warranted. The use of AVP may be justified as an adjuvant in patients not responsive to norepinephrine alone. Dopamine at high doses is associated with larger risk of ischemia and arrhythmia and offers no advantage over norephinephrine. Other vasoconstrictors offer no additional advantages, are less or equally effective, and have a worse safety profile.

In practice, patients will benefit from a highly individualized combination of drugs, such that dobutamine will be chosen for the patient requiring inotropic support, whereas norepinephrine will be preferred to manage the patient with hypotension and vasodilation, or a combination of both in the patient requiring inotropic support and vasopressor therapy.

Vasodilators and atrial natriuretic peptide

Fenoldopam, a selective A-1 dopamine receptor agonist in the kidney, has been recommended for the prophylaxis of AKI post-cardiac surgery. Three randomized controlled trials (RCTs) have shown mixed results. There is no evidence of benefit when used to avoid contrast-induced (CIAKI).

Given the scant evidence of benefit, the use of Theophylline to prevent CIAKI, cannot be recommended on a routine basis. Other phosphodiesterase inhibitors such as levosiendan and enoximone have shown promising results including renal protection in small studies.

Atrial natriuretic peptides (ANP) induce afferent arteriolar dilatation and efferent vasoconstriction as well as increased renal perfusion, diuresis, and natriuresis. Unfortunately, these agents have not shown to be able to avoid the development of AKI; despite promising animal studies, RCTs have shown inconsistent clinical benefit. Atrial natriuretic peptides may be associated with improved outcomes when used in low doses to prevent AKI and in manage postsurgery AKI and should be further explored in those settings. There were no significant adverse events in the prevention studies; however, in the high-dose ANP treatment, there were significant episodes of hypotension and arrhythmia.

Other medications

Multiple trials have studied the use of N-acetyl-cysteine (NAC) for prophylaxis of contrast-induced AKI or other forms of AKI in critically ill patients. Benefit has been limited to intermediate endpoints, but there was no clinically relevant benefit in endpoints such as need for RRT, length of stay, or death. Due to conflicting results, possible adverse reactions and better alternatives, the use of N-acetyl-cysteine has not been recommended for AKI prophylaxis. Other antioxidants such as vitamin C and E and selenium have been suggested but have not demonstrated efficacy.

Mannitol

Mannitol (D-mannitol, $C_6H_{14}O_6$, MW 182 Dalton) is a polysaccharide used for many years to prevent acute kidney injury (AKI). Its purported benefits include intravascular volume expansion, promotion of osmotic diuresis, decreased renal tubular sodium and water resorption, and scavenging of pro-inflammatory reactive oxygen radicals. Current evidence supports the use of mannitol in only a few specific situations including post-renal transplantation.

Mannitol is still used for the management of intracranial hypertension. There is lack of evidence of benefit for other indications. Mannitol use can be associated with significant toxicity including the induction of AKI due to osmotic nephrosis.

Diuretics

Diuretics—including loop diuretics—are not recommended to prevent or ameliorate AKI. To date, four RCTs and three meta-analyses have examined the role of diuretics in established AKI. These studies showed no demonstrable benefit and emphasized the risk of inducing extrarenal injury including hearing loss.

In patients with oliguric AKI, commonly attributed to a more severe degree of renal injury, clinicians often attempt to restore diuresis to control fluid overload expecting that the conversion to nonoliguric AKI will improve patient outcome. Evidence does not support this belief; in the setting of AKI, response to diuretics only indicates a lesser severity of injury. Use of diuretics does not improve renal functional outcomes or survival.

The use of diuretics should be limited to the goals of optimizing fluid management whenever possible, and to help manage electrolyte disorders including hyperkalemia, hypermagnesemia and hypercalcemia. In severe AKI, loop diuretics are generally the only diuretic medications effective, but in some cases the association with thiazides has been shown useful to overcome diuretic resistance.

Pharmacology

This section will emphasize issues of particular relevance to the critically ill patient with AKI.

Normally, the thick ascending loop of Henle (TALH) reabsorbs about 25 percent, and the distal convoluted tubule (DCT) 10 percent of a filtered sodium load. Loop diuretics block the $Na^+K^+2Cl^-$ transporter in the TALH, leading to greater sodium delivery to the distal nephron. Thiazides exert their effect by blocking the electro neutral Na^+/Cl^- transporter in the DCT. Because of the larger fraction of sodium reabsorbed in the TALH, loop diuretic action results in larger sodium and water loss than thiazide diuretics. Moreover, although loop diuretics block tubulo-glomerular feedback, thiazide diuretics enhance this mechanism and, therefore, cause a sharper reduction of glomerular filtration rate (GFR).

Loop diuretics must be present inside the renal tubule to exert their effects. They reach their site of action by filtration and active tubular secretion by organic acid transporters. Their high degree of protein binding (>95 percent) limits their filterability. Half of an administered dose of furosemide reaches the urine unchanged; the other half is metabolized in the kidney by glucurono-conjugation.

The dose-response curve of loop diuretics is sigmoid-shaped. In healthy persons, the steep portion of the curve is at a dose of 40 mg of furosemide, and results in the excretion of 200–250 mM of sodium and 3–4 L water in 4 hours. Forty mg of furosemide, 1 mg of bumetanide, and 20 mg of torsemide are dose equivalents.

The curve is shifted to the right in renal disease, and thus higher doses are necessary to achieve effect: when GFR =15 ml/min, only 10–20 percent is secreted into the tubule. In patients with severe renal dysfunction, maximum effective doses are 160–200 mg or equivalent doses of bumetanide or torsemide. Higher doses should be avoided, as they only increase toxic side effects without much increase in efficacy. This is especially true for furosemide: since it is predominantly metabolized in the kidney, higher doses in renal failure patients lead to prolonged high blood levels and increased risk of ototoxicity.

In contrast to furosemide, the advantages of torsemide and bumetanide include greater potency (five and three times, respectively), and longer half-life. Different loop diuretics also differ in their metabolic pathways: whereas furosemide is predominantly glucuronidated in the kidney, bumetanide and torsemide are metabolized in the liver via the Cytochrome P450 pathway. Because 75 percent of torsemide metabolism is hepatic, its half-life is prolonged in liver-failure patients.

Special problems and questions in the use of diuretics in AKI

1. Co-administration of loop diuretics and albumin

Edematous and hypoalbuminemic patients with anasarca due to liver disease or nephrotic syndrome or severe sepsis associated with multiple organ failure often demonstrate resistance to high dose diuretic administration. Such resistance is due to multiple mechanisms including decreased RBF and GFR, increased volume of distribution of the drug, and decreased bioavailability, binding to urinary albumin, decreased tubular sensitivity, and increased renal glucurono-conjugation.

The efficacy of the albumin-loop diuretic combination is questionable; its effectiveness may be due primarily to extracellular volume expansion leading to improved RBF and GFR and tubular delivery of the drug.

2. Diuretic resistance is due to three main mechanisms:
1. Braking phenomenon due partly to increased intrarenal renin and stimulation of the sympathetic system causing intrarenal vasoconstriction and increased sodium reabsorption.
2. Distal convoluted tubule hypertrophy. It can often be overcome by the addition of thiazide diuretics, but at the price of enhanced tubuloglomerular feedback and worsened GFR.
3. Furosemide short half-life; the problem can be overcome either by using longer half-life loop diuretics (see earlier) or administering the drug by continuous infusion.

3. Adverse effects of diuretic therapy
Volume depletion, hypotension, decreased cardiac output, and worsening renal function are well-known adverse effects. Additionally, diuretics often induce electrolyte depletion, hyponatremia, potassium depletion and metabolic alkalosis and hypomagnesemia, which can lead to cardiac arrhythmia.

Neurohormonal activation including the sympathetic system and renin-angiotensin-aldosterone system is especially troublesome in patients with cardio-renal syndrome.

In the setting of impaired renal function, loop diuretics are not without hazards, including transient episodes of tinnitus, vertigo, or decreased hearing. Furosemide doses should not exceed 1000 mg/day and should preferably remain within the 160–200 mg/day range.

Conclusions

To prevent AKI, main measures include prompt resuscitation of the circulation with fluids, inotropics, vasoconstrictors, and/or vasodilators. Although volume expansion is recommended to avoid the onset of AKI whenever hypovolemia is suspected, uncontrolled volume expansion causes more harm than benefit. Once the patient is adequately volume expanded, judicious use of vasoconstrictors with the goal of raising mean blood pressure to equal or greater than 60 mmHg is adequate, but goals must be individually titrated. Vasodilators may be helpful to manage the patient with severe cardiac dysfunction or hypertension. Some vasodilators may be beneficial to avoid the onset of AKI.

In the critically ill patient, persistent fluid overload must be avoided. It does not benefit the patient and there is evidence of harm.

In the septic patient, *early* volume expansion seems to be beneficial. Beyond that time, fluid overload is associated with worse outcomes in multiple disparate studies.

Use of diuretics should be only short term as long as it is effective, generally at high doses of 160–200 mg, while avoiding utilization of nephrotoxins such as aminoglycosides. Multiple RCT have shown no benefit in the use of diuretics to either prevent or treat established AKI.

If fluid overload must be managed and the patient does not respond to diuretics, persistent use of these drugs will only lead to delay in the initiation of dialysis or ultrafiltration and negative outcomes. In that setting, early initiation of renal replacement therapy may be preferable.

Suggested readings

Bellomo R, Wan L, May C. Vasoactive drugs and acute kidney injury. *Crit Care Med.* 2008;36:S179–S186.

Cerda J, Sheinfeld G, Ronco C. Fluid overload in critically ill patients with acute kidney injury. *Blood Purification.* 2010;29:11–18.

Dellinger RP, Levy MM, Carlet JM, et al. Surviving Sepsis Campaign: International guidelines for management of severe sepsis and septic shock: 2008. *Crit Care Med.* 2008;36:296–327.

Gibney N, Cerda J, Davenport A, et al. Volume management by renal replacement therapy in acute kidney injury. *Int J Artif Organs.* 2008;31:145–155.

Gordon AC, Russell JA, Walley KR, et al. The effects of vasopressin on acute kidney injury in septic shock. *Intensive Care Med.* 2010;36:83–91.

Joannidis M, Druml W, Forni LG, et al. Prevention of acute kidney injury and protection of renal function in the intensive care unit. Expert opinion of the Working Group for Nephrology, ESICM. *Intensive Care Med.* 2010;36:392–411.

Kellum JA, Cerda J, Kaplan LJ, et al. Fluids for prevention and management of acute kidney injury. *Int J Artif Organs.* 2008;31:96–110.

Kellum JA, Pinsky MR. Use of vasopressor agents in critically ill patients. *Curr Opin Crit Care.* 2002;8:236–241.

Mehta RL, Cantarovich F, Shaw A, Hoste E, et al. Pharmacologic approaches for volume excess in acute kidney injury (AKI). *Int J Artif Organs.* 2008;31:127–144.

Patel GP, Grahe JS, Sperry M, et al. Efficacy and safety of dopamine versus norepinephrine in the management of septic shock. *Shock.* 2010;33:375–380.

Russell JA, Walley KR, Singer J, et al. Vasopressin versus norepinephrine infusion in patients with septic shock. *N Engl J Med.* 2008;358:877–887.

Chapter 8

Drug dosing in kidney disease

Thomas D. Nolin and Kristine S. Schonder

Optimal use of drugs in patients with kidney disease (KD), particularly those with superimposed critical illness, requires an awareness of likely pharmacokinetic alterations present, drugs with specific properties lending to their preferred use or contraindications, and drug dosing and adjustment strategies. Kidney disease impacts virtually all aspects of pharmacokinetics, or drug disposition, in the body. These include drug absorption from the administration site, distribution into various body compartments, and clearance from the body. Drug clearance is comprised primarily of nonrenal metabolism and transport, and renal excretion of parent drug and metabolites.

Pharmacokinetics

Absorption

The extent of absorption from an extravascular site of drug administration into the systemic circulation is influenced by numerous factors that ultimately determine a drug's bioavailability (i.e., the fraction of administered dose reaching the systemic circulation). A common cause of low oral bioavailability is drug loss due to its "first-pass" through the intestine and liver, where a drug may be excreted unchanged in the bile or metabolized before entering the systemic circulation. A drug's absorption profile and bioavailability may be altered in patients with KD because of pathophysiological changes in the gastrointestinal tract (GIT), including delayed gastric emptying caused by gastroparesis. Typically, changes in motility slow absorption and affect the time required to reach the maximal plasma concentration, but not the extent of absorption (i.e., maximal plasma concentrations achieved) and bioavailability. However, elevated gastric pH and concurrent drug administration have been associated with reduced bioavailability. High urea concentrations may result in conversion of urea to ammonia by gastric urease. The resulting increase in gastric pH may alter the dissolution or ionization properties of a drug, leading to changes in bioavailability. Antacids, histamine H_2-receptor antagonists, and proton-pump–inhibiting agents also may modify bioavailability by affecting gastric pH and/

or gut motility. Additionally, the ingestion of dairy products, antacids, vitamin supplements, and other sources of cationic molecules may dramatically reduce the bioavailability of some drugs by the formation of insoluble salts or metal ion chelates. Generally, this can be avoided by administering them at least two hours apart from one another. Edema of the GIT also has been cited as a potential cause of altered drug absorption.

Distribution

The extent of drug distribution throughout the body is quantified as the drug's volume of distribution (V_D), the pharmacokinetic term relating the amount of drug in the body to the measured plasma concentration. It does not represent an actual anatomic volume. It is a reflection of the apparent volume of plasma in which a given dose would have to be distributed to achieve the observed plasma concentration. Primary determinants of V_D include plasma protein binding, tissue binding, and total body water, all of which may be altered in the presence of KD:

- Alterations in protein binding can have clinical implications because protein binding determines the free-fraction or fraction of drug that is not protein bound, which, in turn, represents the pharmacologically active moiety. Protein binding also constrains drug distribution because only unbound or free drug crosses cellular membranes.

  - Albumin is the primary binding site for acidic drugs. Protein binding of many acidic drugs, including penicillins, cephalosporins, aminoglycosides, furosemide, and phenytoin, is reduced in patients with KD. The decrease in binding typically is attributed to hypoalbuminemia, qualitative changes in the conformation of the protein-binding site, and/or competition for binding sites by other drugs and metabolites.

  - α1-acid glycoprotein (AAG) is the primary binding site for basic drugs. α1-acid glycoprotein is an acute phase reactant, so concentrations may increase during and after physiologic stress, leading to increased protein binding of basic drugs such as meperidine, propranolol, and lidocaine. Generally, however, binding of basic drugs to AAG appears to be unaffected in patients with KD.

  - Changes in protein binding may result in alterations in V_D, but typically will not have significant clinical implications. This is because an increase in the free fraction may result in increased V_D and hepatic or renal clearance, thereby resulting in a net effect of no significant change in drug exposure.

- Altered tissue binding and total-body-water content also may affect V_D in patients with KD. However, like protein binding, changes in tissue binding probably are irrelevant for the majority of drugs. One exception is digoxin, the V_D of which is decreased by up to 50 percent in patients with severe (stage 5) CKD (i.e., glomerular filtration rate ≤15 mL/min), leading to elevated serum concentrations. Last, hydrophilic compounds would be expected to have an increased V_D in patients with KD because of fluid retention reflected by an increase in extracellular fluid volume, which results in reduced serum concentrations.

Metabolism

Enzymatic metabolism or biotransformation by organs such as the liver and intestine serves to convert drugs through various metabolic pathways to more hydrophilic metabolites, which can then be excreted by the kidneys. Hepatic metabolism of drugs is primarily dependent on hepatic blood flow, enzyme activity, and protein binding:

- Altered hepatic blood flow may affect drug metabolism by increasing or decreasing the rate of drug delivery to the liver. This is most likely to impact drugs whose metabolism is so high that hepatic blood flow and delivery to the liver becomes the rate-limiting step in hepatic clearance. These drugs are called "high extraction ratio" or "blood-flow limited" drugs, and are relatively unaffected by changes in protein binding or hepatic enzyme activity. Conditions that change cardiac output or blood-flow distribution (i.e., sepsis, hypovolemic shock, heart failure, KD) can result in altered drug metabolism of high- extraction-ratio drugs such as lidocaine and beta-blockers.

- In addition to changes in blood flow, KD influences the hepatic clearance of drugs by causing alterations in the intrinsic metabolic activity of selected microsomal enzymes. Drug metabolism occurs primarily via two enzyme pathways: Phase I functional reactions (e.g., oxidation, reduction, hydrolysis) and Phase II conjugation reactions (e.g., glucuronidation, acetylation, sulfation). Cytochrome P450 (CYP) enzymes are responsible for the overwhelming majority of Phase I metabolism. KD has been shown to reduce CYP activity, as well as the activity of several Phase II pathways. As depicted in Table 8.1, the metabolic clearance of numerous drugs is affected by KD.

- In addition to the issues discussed previously under "Distribution," protein-binding changes can alter hepatic clearance of low-extraction-ratio drugs because metabolism is limited to non-protein-bound drug. The extent of metabolism of these drugs is proportional to the fraction unbound. Examples include fentanyl, diltiazem, verapamil, erythromycin, haloperidol, and propofol.

Excretion

Kidney function is the most predictable and quantifiable determinant of drug clearance from the body. Reduction in kidney mass, the number of functioning nephrons, renal blood flow, glomerular filtration rate (GFR), and the rate of tubular secretion account for the decreased renal excretory capacity observed in KD.

Many drugs are renally excreted and require dosage adjustments in KD in order to avoid toxicity (Table 8.1). Drug dosage adjustments are typically based on an individual's kidney function (i.e., glomerular filtration rate [GFR]). Glomerular filtration rate is easily estimated based on age, sex, race, and serum creatinine concentration. This must be done with caution in older adults, critically ill patients, and others with abnormal muscle mass, however. Serum creatinine is a by-product of muscle that is almost completely excreted by the kidneys, so it is an excellent endogenous marker of kidney function. In normal young and healthy individuals, a decline in kidney function results in a predictable rise in

Table 8.1 Effect of decreased kidney function on selected drugs

Drug class/ drugs	Bioavailability	Hepatic Metabolism	Renal Clearance	Volume of distribution	Clinical implications
Anticoagulants					
Low-molecular-weight heparins					
Enoxaparin	N/A	Unchanged	Decreased	Unchanged	Increase dosing interval for CLcr < 30 mL/min Monitor antifactor Xa (anti-Xa) levels
Dalteparin, tinzaparin	N/A	Unchanged	Decreased	Unchanged	No dosage adjustment necessary for CLcr < 30 mL/min Dosing undefined for CLcr < 15 mL/min Monitor antifactor Xa (anti-Xa) levels
Thrombin inhibitors					
Bivalirudin	N/A	Unchanged	Decreased	N/A	Decrease rate of infusion for CLcr < 30 mL/min
Desirudin	N/A	Unchanged	Decreased	N/A	Decrease dose by 66 percent for CLcr < 60mL/min Decrease dose by 90 percent for CLcr < 15mL/min
Fondaparinux	N/A	Unchanged	Decreased	N/A	Renal dosing undefined; Decrease dose for CLcr < 50 mL/min
Lepirudin	N/A	Unchanged	Decreased	N/A	Decrease bolus dose and rate of infusion for CLcr < 60 mL/min Do not administer infusion for CLcr < 15 mL/min or HD (consider alternative)
Warfarin	Unchanged	Decreased	Unchanged	Increased	Decreased binding to albumin increases unbound fraction Monitor INR
Antimicrobials					
Acyclovir	Unchanged	Unchanged	Decreased	Unchanged	Decrease dose and/or increase dosing interval with CLcr < 25 mL/min

Drug					Notes
Aminoglycosides	N/A	Unchanged	Decreased	Unchanged	Increase dosing interval with KD Avoid use with chronic KD
Carbepenems	N/A	Unchanged	Decreased	Unchanged	Decrease dose and/or increase dosing interval with CLcr < 50 mL/min Administer dose after HD
Cephalosporins	Unchanged	Unchanged	Decreased	Decreased	Decrease dose and/or increase dosing interval with CLcr < 30 mL/min Deceased albumin binding can increase free fraction of drug Administer dose after HD
Fluconazole	Unchanged	Unchanged	Decreased	Unchanged	Decrease dose with CLcr < 30 mL/min Administer dose after HD
Fluoroquinolones	Unchanged	Unchanged	Decreased	Unchanged	Decrease maintenance doses (administer loading dose) Administration with cations (antacids, calcium, iron) can decrease absorption via chelation in GI tract Moxifloxacin not affected by KD
Ganciclovir	Unchanged	Unchanged	Decreased	Unchanged	Decrease dose and/or increase dosing interval with CLcr < 60 mL/min
Itraconazole	Unchanged	Unchanged	Unchanged	Unchanged	Avoid use of IV with CLcr < 30 mL/min (solubilizing agent accumulates)
Penicillins	Unchanged	Unchanged	Decreased	Unchanged	Decrease dose and/or increase dosing interval with CLcr < 30 mL/min Deceased albumin binding can increase free fraction of drug Administer dose after HD
Vancomycin	Unchanged	Unchanged	Decreased	Increased	Increase dosing interval with KD
Voriconazole	Unchanged	Unchanged	Unchanged	Unchanged	Avoid use of IV with CLcr < 30 mL/min (solubilizing agent accumulates)

(continued)

Table 8.1 (Continued)

Drug class/drugs	Bioavailability	Hepatic Metabolism	Renal Clearance	Volume of distribution	Clinical implications
Benzodiazepines					
Diazepam	Unchanged	Decreased	Unchanged	Decreased	Monitor for increased CNS effects
Lorazepam	Unchanged	Unchanged	Unchanged	Unchanged	Polyethylene glycol (solubilizing agent) can accumulate with prolonged use in KD
Cardiovascular agents					
ACE- inhibitors	Unchanged	Unchanged	Decreased	Unchanged	Decrease dose for CLcr < 30 mL/min Administer dose after HD Fosinopril is not affected by altered kidney function
Beta-blockers					
Atenolol	Unchanged	Unchanged	Decreased	Unchanged	Decrease dose for CLcr < 30 mL/min Removed by HD (administer supplemental dose)
Nadolol	Unchanged	Unchanged	Decreased	Unchanged	Increase dosing interval with CLcr < 50 mL/min
Propranolol	Unchanged	Unchanged	Unchanged	Decreased	Increased protein binding with uremia decreases free fraction of drug Decreased effectiveness
Sotalol	Unchanged	Unchanged	Decreased	Unchanged	Increase dosing interval with CLcr < 60 mL/min Avoid use with CLcr < 40 mL/min
Digoxin	Unchanged	Unchanged	Decreased	Decreased	Decrease dose or increase dosing interval with CLcr < 50 mL/min

Diuretics				
Loop diuretics	Decreased at site of action	Unchanged	Decreased	Decreased	Increase dose required to increase availability at site of action Combination with thiazide diuretics useful to overcome resistance Deceased albumin binding can increase free fraction of drug
Thiazide diuretics	Decreased at site of action	Unchanged	Decreased	Unchanged	Increase dose required to increase availability at site of action
H_2-receptor antagonists	Unchanged	Unchanged	Decreased	Unchanged	Decrease dose and/or increase dosing interval with CLcr < 30 mL/min
Insulin	Unchanged	Unchanged	Decreased	Unchanged	Decrease dose with KD Increase dosing interval with long-acting insulin products
Ketorolac	Unchanged	Unchanged	Decreased	Unchanged	Decrease dose or increase dosing interval with KD Avoid use with advanced KD
Morphine	Unchanged	Decreased	Decreased	Increased	Volume overload increases distribution and decreased serum concentrations Decreased renal clearance decreases elimination—can lead to neurologic impairment
Phenytoin	Unchanged	Decreased	Unchanged	Increased	Monitor free drug concentration Deceased albumin binding can increase free fraction of drug

ACE—angiotensin converting enzyme; CLcr—creatinine clearance; HD—hemodialysis; KD- kidney disease serum creatinine concentration. However, because muscle mass decreases with age and during critical illness, creatinine production and presence in the serum also decreases, so the serum creatinine value may not accurately reflect the true level of kidney function.

Renally excreted drugs requiring dosage adjustments include numerous antimicrobials, digoxin, lithium, and antiulcer medications like famotidine and ranitidine. Many drugs also require dose adjustment because of the production of active metabolites that are renally eliminated. These include allopurinol, morphine, meperidine, propoxyphene, and procainamide (Table 8.2).

Drug selection

Drug selection for the critically ill patient with KD requires careful consideration of the pharmacokinetic and overall pharmacodyanamic effects of the drug. For a given therapeutic problem, certain drugs and drug classes may be preferred in the patient with KD.

Analgesics

The lipid-soluble nature of most opiates decreases the effect of kidney failure on the pharmacokinetic properties of the parent drug compound. However, meperidine, morphine, codeine, and propoxyphene are metabolized in the liver to biologically active compounds that are extensively cleared by the kidneys and can accumulate in KD and lead to substantial toxicities (Table 8.2). Fentanyl is the preferred opioid agent for management of analgesia in the critically ill patient with KD. Hydromorphone may be used with caution at lower doses, as the inactive metabolite can accumulate with kidney failure.

Nonsteroidal anti-inflammatory agents (NSAIDs) have increased potential to cause acute changes in kidney function in patients with poor renal perfusion. Ketorolac is eliminated by the kidney and requires dosage adjustment in KD.

Anticoagulants

Heparin binding to albumin is decreased in KD, resulting in a higher V_D. Clinically, however, no effect is observed on prothrombin time. Low-molecular weight heparins are eliminated by the kidneys and can have prolonged half-lives in patients with KD requiring dosage adjustments. Dosage adjustments are outlined for enoxaparin for patients with KD (Table 8.1). Dalteparin or tinzaparin may be preferred in patients with creatinine clearance (CLcr) < 30 mL/min, but there are no defined dosing strategies for CLcr < 15 mL/min. Likewise, the thrombin inhibitors dabigatran, bivalrudin, desirudin, fondaparinux, and lepirudin are renally eliminated and require dosage adjustments for KD. Argatroban is the preferred thrombin inhibitor for patients with KD.

Antimicrobials

Beta-lactam antibiotics are excreted via the kidneys and require dosage adjustments in patients with KD. Other antimicrobials that are extensively eliminated

Table 8.2 Drugs with active metabolites that may accumulate in patients with decreased kidney function

Drug	Metabolite(s)	Pharmacologic activity of metabolite(s)	Clinical implications
Acebutolol	Diacetolol	Beta-blockade	Decrease dose to 50% of normal dose for CLcr < 50 mL/min; decrease dose to 25% of normal dose for CLcr < 10 mL/min
Allopurinol	Oxypurinol	Bone marrow suppression	Decrease dose to 50% of normal dose for CLcr < 50 mL/min
Codeine	Norcodeine; codeine-6-glucuronide; morphine	Hypotension; CNS depression; respiratory depression	Decrease dose to 75% of normal dose for CLcr 10–50 mL/min; decrease dose to 50% of normal dose for CLcr < 10 mL/min
Meperidine	Normeperidine	CNS stimulation; seizure	Avoid use with advanced or severe KD
Midazolam	Alpha-hydroxy-midazolam	Sedation	Decrease dose to 50% of normal dose for CLcr < 10 mL/min
Morphine	Morphine-3-glucuronide; morphine-6-glucuronide	Analgesia; CNS and respiratory depression	Metabolite is has 10 times activity of parent compound
			Decreased dose to 75% of normal dose for CLcr < 50 mL/min; decrease dose to 50% of normal dose for CLcr < 10 mL/min
Procainamide	N-acetyl-procainamide	Antiarrhythmic activity	Use with caution in KD
Propoxyphene	Norpropoxyphene	Sedation; hypoglycemia; cardiovascular toxicity	Use with caution in KD

by the kidneys include fluoroquinolones (with the exception of moxifloxacin), the antivirals acyclovir and ganciclovir, aminoglycosides, vancomycin, and the antifungal fluconazole. All of these drugs require dosage adjustments in patients with KD. Itraconazole and voriconazole are extensively metabolized in the liver and do not require dosage adjustments for KD. However, the IV formulations of each are prepared with solubilizing agents that are eliminated via the kidney and can accumulate in KD. Therefore, the IV formulations of both drugs should be avoided in patients with CLcr < 30 mL/min.

Cardiovascular agents

As a drug class, ACE-inhibitors are eliminated via the kidney and require dosage adjustments for CLcr < 30 mL/min. Some beta-blockers, including atenolol, nadolol, and sotalol, are eliminated via the kidneys and require dosing adjustments for KD. The protein binding of propranolol is increased in KD, which decreases the effectiveness of the drug. Digoxin dosing is complicated in KD because of the decrease in the V_D and decreased renal elimination.

Diuretics

Both loop and thiazide diuretics have decreased effect in patients with KD because of decreased penetration into the kidney at the site of action. Loop diuretics generally require higher doses for effect in KD. Thiazide diuretics are considered to be ineffective with CLcr < 30 mL/min, but they are useful as adjunctive agents to increase the effects of loop diuretics.

Sedatives

Both the hepatic metabolism and V_D of diazepam are decreased in patients with KD, which can increase the sedative effects. Midazolam is metabolized in the liver to compounds with substantial pharmacologic activity and avoided in patients with severe KD because of the prolonged sedative effects. Lorazepam may be preferred for short-term use in patients with KD, but prolonged use can result in accumulation of polyethylene glycol, which can worsen kidney function. Propofol or dexmedetomidine are alternative agents for patients with KD.

Other considerations

Phenytoin exhibits complicated pharmacokinetics in patients with KD because of decreased protein binding, increased V_D, and decreased hepatic metabolism in patients with KD. Free phenytoin concentrations should be used to monitor therapeutic efficacy in patients with KD.

H_2-receptor blockers are renally eliminated and can accumulate in patients with KD, requiring dosage adjustments. Proton-pump inhibitors (PPIs) may be preferred in patients with severe KD.

Drug dosing and adjustment strategies

The primary objective in adjusting drug dosing regimens in patients with kidney disease is typically to maintain the same average unbound drug concentrations in plasma that would be observed in patients with normal kidney function, thereby maintaining similar safety and efficacy. Several strategies are available for this purpose:

• Use of FDA-approved dosing recommendations or guidelines when available are strongly encouraged. Nomograms may be used to adjust the dose of drugs that are predominantly eliminated renally on the premise that their total-body clearance and renal clearance are proportional to kidney function (i.e., creatinine clearance). For example, after calculating creatinine clearance, nomograms may be used to determine the appropriate dosing interval for a given level of kidney function. It must be noted, however, that secondary sources of drug information should be cross-checked with one another because significant variability in recommendations are known to exist.

- When possible, individualized dosing based on plasma concentrations should be used in lieu of nomograms. Therapeutic drug monitoring incorporating prospective PK techniques are preferred to achieve desired plasma concentrations for drugs with narrow therapeutic ranges or target plasma concentrations, such as aminoglycosides and vancomycin.

- In general, drug dosage adjustments are not necessary until a patient's kidney function declines to ≤ 50 percent of normal (i.e., CLcr ≤ 60 mL/min, or stages 3–5 CKD). There are two primary methods of dose adjustment commonly utilized in patients receiving intermittent dosing, both of which assume no change in other PK parameters such as bioavailability, protein binding, volume of distribution, and nonrenal clearance. These assumptions are rarely valid in patients with kidney disease, especially those with superimposed critical illness.

  - The first approach is to maintain the normal individual dose and extend the dosing interval such that the dose is administered less frequently. This is most commonly utilized in patients with KD and is preferred with drugs that require target peak or trough serum concentrations, such as aminoglycosides or vancomycin.

  - The alternative approach commonly used is to reduce the individual dose administered and maintain the normal dosing frequency. This results in peak and trough concentrations that are closer together than the preceding alternative approach, and is preferred with drugs that require maintenance of serum concentrations over a dosing interval, such as beta-lactam antibiotics.

  - Some drugs, such as fluoroquinolones, may require a combination of both strategies in severe KD: reducing the individual dose and extending the dosing interval.

- For patients receiving drugs via continuous intravenous infusion, a change in renal clearance of a drug attributed to reduced kidney function is compensated by a corresponding proportional reduction in the dosing or infusion rate. For example, a 75 percent reduction in kidney function would require a similar decrease in the infusion rate (i.e., to 25 percent the usual rate) in order to achieve normal serum drug concentrations.

- A loading dose is sometimes indicated when it is clinically important to rapidly achieve target serum concentrations of a drug. This is particularly vital when the drug's renal clearance is decreased and corresponding half-life is significantly increased, thereby extending the time required to achieve steady state serum concentrations. Loading doses are generally unchanged in patients with kidney disease compared to those with normal kidney function. Exceptions include digoxin and phenytoin, as mentioned previously.

Suggested readings

Aronoff GR, Bennett WM, Berns JS, et al. (Eds). *Drug prescribing in renal failure: Dosing guidelines for adults and children.* 5th ed. Philadelphia: American College of Physicians, 2007.

Boucher BA, Wood GC, Swanson JM. Pharmacokinetic changes in critical illness. *Crit Care Clin.* 2006;22:255–271.

Brater DC. Drug dosing in patients with impaired renal function. *Clin Pharmacol Ther.* 2009;86:483–489.

Gabardi S, Abramson S. Drug dosing in chronic kidney disease. *Med Clin North Am.* 2005;89:649–687.

Nolin TD, Frye RF, Matzke GR. Hepatic drug metabolism and transport in patients with kidney disease. *Am J Kidney Dis.* 2003;42:906–925.

Power BM, Forbes AM, van Heerden PV, et al. Pharmacokinetics of drugs used in critically ill adults. *Clin Pharmacokinet.* 1998;34:25–56.

Verbeeck RK, Musuamba FT. Pharmacokinetics and dosage adjustment in patients with renal dysfunction. *Eur J Clin Pharmacol.* 2009;65:757–773.

Chapter 9

Renal replacement therapy (RRT) indications, timing, and patient selection

John A. Kellum

Indications for RRT

Indications for renal replacement therapy (RRT) fall into two broad categories, so-called "renal" (i.e., to specifically address the consequences of renal failure) and "nonrenal" (without necessitating renal failure). Although the distinction is not always precise, it is a reasonably easy way to categorize indications for RRT.

Renal indications

The manifestations of acute kidney disease (as discussed in chapter 1) and summarized in Table 9.1 include oliguria, (leading to volume overload), azotemia (leading to a host of clinical complications), hyperkalemia, and metabolic acidosis. Although there is no consensus regarding the precise level of dysfunction in any of these areas that should prompt initiation of RRT, general agreement exists on the following:

General indications for RRT
Volume overload (e.g., pulmonary edema).
Azotemia with uremic symptoms.
Hyperkalemia (>6.0 mmol/l).
Metabolic acidosis (pH <7.2) due to renal failure.

Volume overload
Volume overload usually occurs in the setting of oliguria, but it may occur simply because urine output is insufficient to maintain fluid balance in the face of large volume input—even if true oliguria is not present. Furthermore, most authorities recommend therapy before volume overload becomes clinically manifest and thus RRT may be used to "create space" for additional fluids (e.g., nutritional support, antibiotics) that are scheduled to be administered.

Table 9.1 Manifestations of renal failure

System	Complication(s)	Mechanism(s)	Clinical features
Cardiovascular	Volume overload	Salt/water retention	Edema, heart failure, hypertension
Electrolyte and Acid-Base	Hyponatremia, hyperkalemia, acidosis, azotemia	Impaired free water excretion, chloride accumulation	Hypotension, impaired glucose metabolism, decreased muscle protein synthesis, cardiac dysrhythmias
Gastrointestinal	Impaired nutrient absorption, GI bleeding, abdominal compartment syndrome	Bowel edema, platelet dysfunction, volume overload	Nausea, vomiting, decreased mucosal/ intestinal absorption, increased intra-abdominal pressures
Hematological	Anemia, platelet dysfunction	Decreased erythropoietin, decreased von Wilibrand's factor	Anemia, bleeding
Immune	Infections, Immune suppression	Impaired neutrophil function	Infection, sepsis
Nervous	Encephalopathy	Uremic toxins, hyponatremia	Asterixis, delirium, coma
Respiratory	Pleural effusions, pulmonary edema	Volume overload, decrease oncotic pressure,?direct uremic toxicity	Pleural effusion, pulmonary edema, respiratory failure

There is controversy about the role of diuretics in the setting of volume overload secondary to acute renal failure. Although most clinicians will attempt diuretics prior to initiation of RRT, there is wide variation about how long or intense such a trial will be or how success will be defined. Although it is obviously desirable to avoid RRT, there is little evidence to suggest that diuretics can be successful in achieving this goal and available evidence even suggests potential harm. Importantly, attempts to increase urine output with diuretics should only be directed toward treatment of volume overload or hyperkalemia, not oliguria per se. Large observation studies have failed to show benefit from diuretics in critically ill patients with oliguria and some studies have shown harm.

Diuretic therapy

A loop diuretic such as furosemide is given in a dose of 20–40 mg intravenously. If this dose is ineffective, a higher dose can be tried in 30–60 minutes. Higher doses may be needed if the patient has previously received diuretic therapy. If bolus doses of 80 mg every 6 hours are ineffective, an infusion may be started (1–5 mg/h IV). A thyazide diuretic such as chlorothiazide (250–500 mg IV) or metolazone (10–20 mg PO) can be used in conjunction with a loop diuretic to improve diuresis. In general, there is no point in continuing diuretic therapy if it is not effective; loop diuretics in particular may be nephrotoxic. See Table 9.2. Discontinue all diuretics prior to initiating RRT.

Azotemia

Azotemia, the retention of urea and other nitrogenous waste products, results from a reduction in glomerular filtration rate (GFR) and is a cardinal feature of kidney failure. However, like oliguria, azotemia represents not only disease but also a normal response of the kidney to extracellular volume depletion or a decreased renal blood flow. Conversely, a "normal" GFR in the face of volume depletion could only be viewed as renal dysfunction. Thus, changes in urine output and GFR are neither necessary nor sufficient for the diagnosis of renal pathology. Yet, no simple alternative for the diagnosis currently exists.

Azotemia is also a biochemical marker of the uremic syndrome, a condition caused by a diverse group of toxins that are normally excreted but build up in the circulation and in the tissues during renal failure. The clinical manifestations of the uremic syndrome are shown in the Table 9.1.

Although uremic symptoms correlate with the level of urea in the blood, the relationship between BUN and symptoms is not consistent across individuals or even within a given individual at different times. Thus, there is no threshold level of BUN that defines uremia nor provides a specific indication for RRT. Instead, the provision of RRT and, indeed, decisions about timing and intensity should be individualzed to patients on the basis of clinical factors not solely on the basis of biochemical markers.

Hyperkalemia

Hyperkalemia may be severe and can be life threatening. The risks of hyperkalemia are greatest when it developes rapidly when serum concentrations in excess of 6 mmol/L may produce cardiac dysrythmias. The earliest electocardiographic sign of hyperkalemia is peaking of the T waves. This finding is associated cardiac irritability and should prompt emergent treatment. Temporary management of severe hyperkalemia (while preparing for RRT) include intravenous calcium chloride (10 ml of 10 percent solution) to reduce cardiac irritability and a combination of insulin (10 units IV) and dextrose (50 ml D50) given

Table 9.2 Diuretic dosing

	Oral	IV	Infusion
Metolazone	10–20 mg qd		
Chlorothiazide		250–500 mg IV	
Furosemide	20–40 mg 6–24 hrly	5–80 mg 6–24 hrly	1–10 mg/h
Torsemide	5–20 mg 6–24 hrly	5–20 mg 6–24 hrly	1–5 mg/h
Bumetanide	0.5–1 mg 6–24 hrly	0.5–2 mg 6–24 hrly	1–5 mg/h

together over 20 minutes to shift potassium intracellularly—that is, monitor blood glucose levels.

Metabolic acidosis

Renal failure causes metabolic acidosis by retention of various acid anions (e.g., phosphate, sulfate) as well as from renal tubular dysfunction resulting in hyperchloremic acidosis. Clinical manifestations range from acute alterations in inflammatory cell function to chronic changes in bone mineralization. Mild alterations can be managed using oral sodium bicarbonate or calcium carbonate. RRT is effective in removing acids as well as correcting plasma sodium and chloride balance and is generally targeted at maintaining an arterial pH >7.30 (see Table 9.1).

"Nonrenal" indications

So-called nonrenal indications for RRT are to remove various dialyzable substances from the blood. These substances include drugs, poisons, contrast agents, and cytokines.

Drug and toxin removal

Blood purification techniques have long been used for removal of various dialyzable drugs and toxins. A list of common drugs and toxins that can be readily removed using RRT is shown in Table 9.3. The majority of poisoning cases do not require treatment with RRT. Indeed, the drugs or toxins that are most commonly responsible for poison-related fatalities are not amenable to RRT (e.g., acetaminophen, tricyclic antidepressants, short-acting barbiturates, stimulants, and "street drugs"). In general the size of molecule and the degree of protein binding determines the degree to which the substance can be removed (smaller, non-protein-bound substances are easiest to remove). Continuous renal replacement therapy (CRRT) may be effective in removing substances with higher degrees of protein binding and is sometimes used to remove substances with very long plasma half-lives.

The role of CRRT in the management of acute poisonings is not well established. There is lower drug clearance relative per unit of time compared to intermittent hemodialysis (IHD), but CRRT has a distinct advantage in hemodynamically unstable patients who are unable to tolerate the rapid solute and fluid losses associated with IHD or even other techniques such as hemoperfusion. CRRT may also be effective for the slow, continuous removal of substances with large volumes of distribution, a high degree of tissue binding, or for substances that are prone to "rebound phenomenon" (e.g., lithium, procainamide, and methotrexate). In such cases, CRRT may even be used as adjuvant therapy with IHD or hemoperfusion. See Table 9.3.

Contrast agents

Renal replacement therapy has been used to remove radio-contrast agents for many years, but the purpose of this treatment has changed over time. In the past, ionic, high osmolar contrast was used for imaging studies, and RRT was

Table 9.3 Common poisonings treated with RRT*

Substance	Extracorporeal method	Comments
Methanol	Hemodialysis	RRT should be continued until the serum methanol concentration is < 25 mg/dL and the anion-gap metabolic acidosis and osmolal gap are normal. Rebound may occur up to 36 hrs.
Isopropanol	Hemodialysis	RRT effectively removes isopropanol and acetone, although it is usually unnecessary except in severe cases (prolonged coma, myocardial depression, renal failure).
Ethylene glycol	Hemodialysis	RRT should be continued until the ethylene glycol level is < 20 mg/dL and metabolic acidosis or other signs of systemic toxicity have resolved. Rebound may occur up to 24 hrs.
Lithium	IHD/CRRT	IHD removed lithium faster but rebound is significant problem and can be addressed effectively with CRRT.
Salicylate	IHD/CRRT	Both IHD/CRRT have been reported in the management of salicylate poisoning.
Theophylline	IHD/CRRT/Hemoperfusion	RRT should be continued until clinical improvement and a plasma level < 20 mg/L is obtained. Rebound may occur.
Valproic acid	IHD/CRRT/Hemoperfusion	At supratherapeutic drug levels plasma proteins become saturated, and the fraction of unbound drug increases substantially and becomes dialyzable.

*Note: other treatments are also required for many of these substances

often used to remove these substances, as well as to remove fluid, in patients with renal failure who were at risk for congestive heart failure from the large osmotic load. These patients could not excrete the contrast and would develop pulmonary edema after contrast administration. In more recent years, nonionic, low-osmolality or even iso-osmolar agents have been developed, and the risk of pulmonary edema has decreased significantly. However, all radio-contrast agents are nephrotoxic and CRRT is being advocated by some experts to help prevent so-called contrast nephropathy. Standard intermittent hemodialysis has been shown to remove radio-contrast agents, but it does not appear to prevent contrast nephropathy. Despite less efficiency in removing contrast, CRRT has been shown to result in less contrast nephropathy, particularly when it is begun prior to or in conjunction with contrast administration. However, the effect is controversial and most centers do not currently offer RRT for prevention of contrast nephropathy. See Table 9.4.

Table 9.4 Methods to reduce contrast nephropathy include

	Oral	IV	Dosing*
Saline		0.9 percent (154 mEq/L)	1 ml/kg/hr begun 12 hrs OR 3 ml/kg/hr begun 1 hr prior to procedure AND 1 ml/kg/hr continuing 6 hrs after procedure
NaHCO$_3$ in water		150 mEq/L	1 ml/kg/hr begun 12 hrs OR 3 ml/kg/hr begun 1 hr prior to procedure AND 1 ml/kg/hr continuing 6 hrs after procedure
N-acetylcysteine	1200 mg every 12 hrs	1200 mg every 12 hrs	beginning 24 hrs before and continuing 24 hrs after procedure

Cytokines

Many endogenous mediators of sepsis can be removed using continuous veno-venous hemofiltration (CVVH) or continuous veno venous hemodiafiltration (CVVHDF) (dialysis is not able to remove these mediators). This observation has prompted many investigators to attempt to use CVVH as an adjunctive therapy in sepsis. Although it remains controversial whether CVVH offers additional benefit in patients with renal failure and sepsis, available evidence does not support a role for CVVH for the removal of cytokines in patients without renal failure. If CVVH is capable of removing cytokines, the effect of standard "renal dose" CVVH appears to be small. However, some individuals appear to respond with improved hemodynamics, especially to higher doses of CVVH.

Timing of RRT

When to initiate RRT

The simplest answer to the question, "When should RRT be started?" would be when the indications discussed earlier are met. Numerous attempts have been made to reach a consensus on timing of RRT. The Acute Dialysis Quality Initiative (ADQI) first addressed this issue in 2000 but it was unable to reach consensus beyond stating that a patient is considered to require RRT when he or she has "an acute fall of GFR and has developed, or is at risk of, clinically significant solute imbalance/toxicity or volume overload." In essence, this amounts to saying that RRT should begin when a patient has "symptomatic" acute renal failure. What constitutes symptomatic is a mater of clinical judgment and how one interprets "at risk." Most, but not all, experts advise that RRT should begin *before* clinical complications occur, but it is often difficult to know exactly when such a point occurs. For example, subtle abnormalities in platelet function can begin early in AKI prior to the time when most clinicians would begin RRT.

Observational studies of AKI using RIFLE criteria have provided two important pieces of information: acute renal failure (stage F by RIFLE) is common among critically ill patients (10–20 percent of ICU patients) and is associated with a three- to tenfold increase in the risk of death prior to discharge. Given the profound increase in the risk of death, many investigators have asked why more patients don't receive RRT, yet many patients with acute renal failure recover renal function without ever receiving RRT. Should these patients receive RRT? Current evidence is insufficient to answer this question, but given the low rates of complications associated with CRRT, and high risk of death associated with AKI, consideration should be given to starting therapy early (e.g., when F criteria is present rather than waiting for complications to occur).

When to stop RRT

An even more difficult question to answer than when to start is the when to stop RRT. Again the simplest answer would be "when renal function has recovered," but two problems exist with this simple answer. First, it is not always easy to determine when renal function has recovered and it is also unclear what amount of recovery should be sought prior to cessation of therapy. In essence, the question is not dissimilar to the question about so-called weaning from mechanical ventilation and very little is actually known about how and when "weaning" from RRT should occur. One approach that was used in the largest trial of dialysis intensity published to date, used the following rule:

Assess for recovery of renal function if urine volume >30 mL/hour, 6 hour timed urine collections obtained for assessment of creatinine clearance:

Creatinine clearance	Management of RRT
<12 mL/min	Continue RRT
12–20 mL/min	Clinician judgment
>20 mL/min	Discontinue RRT

Patient Selection for CRRT

Which patients should receive CRRT?

Once the decision is made to initiate RRT, the question of which modality (intermittent versus continuous) arises. The following considerations influence the choice of modality, although, strictly speaking, there are few absolute indications for one modality over the other:

- *Hemodynamic stability:* CRRT is preferred for patients with or at risk for hypotension. In practice, this usually means patients who require vasopressor support either at baseline or as a result of treatment. The ATN trial demonstrated that hypotension is extremely common with intermittent hemodialysis.

- **Intracranial hypertension:** This is an absolute indication for CRRT (over standard intermittent RRT). Intermittent hemodialysis induces much greater fluid shifts and is, therefore, contraindicated in patients with increased intracranial pressure.
- **Severe volume overload and high obligatory fluid intake:** Even in hemodyanamically stable patients, severe volume overload or patients with mild fluid overload but high daily fluid requirements (usually for medications and nutritional support) may be more effectively managed with CRRT. For example, it is unusual to remove more than 3–4 L of volume in a 4-hour dialysis session. Yet it is quite common to remove 200–300 ml/hr (5–7 L per day) or even more with CRRT.
- **Mechanical ventilation:** For patients unable to tolerate weaning trials on nondialysis days, CRRT (or daily dialysis) may be better.
- **High protein turnover/catabolic patients:** For some critically ill patients, it may be difficult to control solute with alternate-day dialysis. Patient with very high pre-dialysis BUN may be better treated with CRRT.
- **Hyperkalemia:** When rapid solute clearance is necessary, such as in severe hyperkalemia, intermittent therapy is generally preferred. Continuos renal replacement therapy is usually quite effective for hyperkalemia, but intermittent therapy will be somewhat faster.

Suggested readings

Hoste EA, Clermont G, Kersten A, et al: RIFLE criteria for acute kidney injury is associated with hospital mortality in critically ill patients: A cohort analysis. *Crit Care.* 2006; 10:R73.

Kellum JA, Mehta RL, Levin A, et al: Development of a clinical research agenda for acute kidney injury using an international, interdisciplinary, three-step modified Delphi process. *Clin J Am Soc Nephrol.* 2008;3:887–894.

Lee PT, Chou KJ, Liu CP, et al: Renal protection for coronary angiography in advanced renal failure patients by prophylactic hemodialysis. A randomized controlled trial. *J Am Coll Cardiol.* 2007;50:1015–1020.

Mehta RL, Pascual MT, Soroko S, et al: Diuretics, mortality, and nonrecovery of renal function in acute renal failure. *JAMA.* 2002;288:2547–2553.

Palevsky PM, Zhang JH, O'Connor TZ, et al: Intensity of Renal Support in Critically Ill Patients with Acute Kidney Injury. *N Engl J Med.* 2008; EPub May 20.

Uchino S, Bellomo R, Morimatsu H, et al: Continuous renal replacement therapy: a worldwide practice survey. *Intensive Care Med.* 2007;33:1563–1570.

Uchino S, Bellomo R, Morimatsu H, et al: Discontinuation of Continuous Renal Replacement Therapy: A Prospective Multi-center Observational study. *Crit Care Med.* 2009;37:2576–2582.

Uchino S, Doig GS, Bellomo R, et al: Diuretics and mortality in acute renal failure. *Crit Care Med.* 2004;32:1669–1677.

Chapter 10

Choosing a renal replacement therapy in acute kidney injury
Technical and clinical considerations

Jorge Cerdá and Claudio Ronco

Most hospital-acquired acute kidney injury (AKI) occurs in the intensive care unit (ICU) and is associated with elevated morbidity and mortality. A recent international survey showed that 80 percent of patients with AKI in the ICU are treated with continuous renal replacement therapy (CRRT), 17 percent with intermittent hemodialysis (IHD) and 3 percent with peritoneal dialysis or SLED.

Newer techniques of renal substitution therapy have allowed a conceptual shift from renal "replacement" to renal "support" therapies, whereby the strategies to treat AKI have become an integral part of the overall critically ill patient management, with "renal" and "nonrenal" applications such as sepsis and acute respiratory distress syndrome (ARDS) (Table 10.1).

Table 10.1 Characteristics of the "ideal" treatment modality of AKI in the ICU
Preserves homeostasis
Does not increase co-morbidity
Does not worsen patient's underlying condition
Is inexpensive
Is simple to manage
Is not burdensome to the ICU staff

From Lameire N, Van Biesen W, Vanholder R. Dialysing the patient with acute renal failure in the ICU: the emperor's clothes? *Nephrol Dial Transplant* 1999;14:2570–2573.

The hemodynamic stability of the critically ill patient is the main determinant of the most appropriate dialysis modality (Table 10.2).

When choosing the modality of renal replacement therapy most appropriate for each patient, multiple considerations must be kept in mind (Table 10.3).

Table 10.2 Indications for specific renal replacement therapies

Therapeutic goal	Hemodynamics	Preferred therapy
Fluid removal	Stable	Intermittent isolated UF
	Unstable	Slow UF
Urea clearance	Stable	Intermittent hemodialysis
	Unstable	CRRT
		Convection: CAVH, CVVH
		Diffusion: CAVHD, CVVHD
		Both: CAVHDF, CVVHDF
Severe hyperkalemia	Stable/Unstable	Intermittent hemodialysis
Severe metabolic acidosis	Stable	Intermittent hemodialysis
	Unstable	CRRT
Severe hyperphosphoremia	Stable/Unstable	CRRT
Brain edema	Unstable	CRRT

From Murray P, Hall J. Renal replacement therapy for acute renal failure. *Am J Respir Crit Care Med.* 2000;162:777–781.

Table 10.3 Considerations in renal replacement therapy for AKI

Consideration	Components	Varieties
Dialysis modality	Intermittent hemodialysis	Daily, every other day, SLED
	Continuous renal replacement therapies	AV, VV
	Peritoneal dialysis	
Dialysis biocompatibility	Membrane characteristics	
Dialyzer performance	Efficiency	
	Flux	
Dialysis delivery	Timing of initiation	Early, late
	Intensity of dialysis	Prescription vs. delivery
	Adequacy of dialysis	Dialysis dose

In addition to the patient's hemodynamic stability, choice between the various renal replacement modalities rests on solute clearance goals, volume control, and anticoagulation (Table 10.4).

The different modalities of CRRT (Figure 10.1) are defined by the main mechanism with which clearance is achieved: simple diffusion (continuous veno venous hemodialysis, CVVHD); convection (continuous hemofiltration, CVVH); or a combination of both (continuous hemodiafiltration, CVVHDF).

These different modalities differ in the magnitude of the clearance achieved by convection or diffusion, the vascular access and the need for fluid replacement (in the case of hemofiltration) (Table 10.5).

The implications of the dose of dialysis on patient outcomes was extensively discussed in chapter 9. Previous reviews have discussed the fundamental operational characteristics of CRRT. Recently, the Acute Dialysis Quality Initiative (ADQI) published a consensus on fluid and volume management, which is relevant to the present discussion.

Arterio-venous or veno-venous blood circuits

Arterio-venous (AV) systems are not used except in emergent situations, when veno-venous (VV) systems are not available. AV system limitations include arterial damage, blood flow dependency on systemic hemodynamics, and insufficient dialysis dose.

Table 10.4 Advantages and disadvantages of various renal replacement modalities

Modality	Use in hemodynamically unstable patients	Solute clearance	Volume control	Anti-coagulation
PD	Yes	++	++	No
IHD	Possible	++++	+++	Yes/no
IHF	Possible	+++	+++	Yes/no
Intermittent IHF	Possible	++++	+++	Yes/no
Hybrid techniques	Possible	++++	++++	Yes/no
CVVH	Yes	+++/++++	++++	Yes/no
CVVHD	Yes	+++/++++	++++	Yes/no
CVVHDF	Yes	++++	++++	Yes/no

HDF: Hemodiafiltration; CVVH: Continuous hemofiltration; CVVHD: Continuous hemodialysis; CVVHDF: Continuous hemodiafiltration; IHD: Intermittenthemodialysis; IHF: Intermittent hemofiltration; PD: Peritoneal dialysis. Modified from Davenport A. Renal replacement therapy in acute kidney injury: Which method to use in the intensive care unit? *Saudi J Kidney Dis Transpl.* 2008;19:529–536.

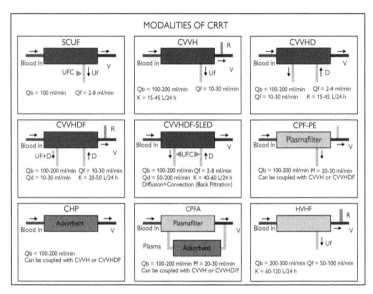

Figure 10.1 Modalities of CRRT. Techniques available today for renal replacement in the intensive care unit.

From Cerda J, Ronco C. Modalities of continuous renal replacement therapy: technical and clinical considerations. Semin Dial. 2009;22:114–122.

CAVH, continuous arterio–venous hemofiltration; CHP, continuous hemoperfusion; CPFA, plasmafiltration coupled with adsorption; CPF-PE, continuous plasmafiltration-plasma exchange; CVVH, continuous veno-venous hemofiltration; CVVHD, continuous veno-venoushemodialysis; CVVHDF, continuous veno-venous hemodiafiltration; CVVHDF, continuous high-flux dialysis; D, dialysate; HVVF, high-volume hemofiltration; K, clearance; Pf, plasmafiltrate flow; Qb, blood flow; Qd, dialysate flow; Qf, ultrafiltration rate; R, replacement; SCUF, slow continuous ultrafiltration; SLEDD, sustained low efficiency daily dialysis; UFC, ultrafiltration control system.

Choice of CRRT modality

- Modality selection for renal support in critically ill patients with acute kidney injury (AKI) is a controversial subject. Both IHD and CRRT are established therapies for such patients.
- Hemodynamic instability and large ongoing solute and fluid removal requirements often render IHD unsuitable at least in the early part of the clinical course, even when performed on a daily basis. The recent ATN (Palevsky, 2008) and RENAL (Bellomo, 2009) trials consolidate the evidence for CRRT and IHD as the established modalities of renal replacement therapy in the ICU.
- Sustained low-efficiency dialysis (SLED), also known as extended daily dialysis (EDD) is a more recently proposed dialysis modality for the AKI population. Evidence on the effect of SLED on patient outcomes is insufficient; this

Table 10.5 Modalities of continuous renal replacement therapy

Technique	Clearance convection	Mechanism diffusion	Vascular access	Fluid replacement
SCUF	+	-	Large vein	0
CAVH	++++	-	Artery and vein	+++
CVVH	++++	-	Large vein	+++
CAVHD	+	++++	Artery and vein	+++
CVVHD	+	++++	Large vein	+/0
CAVHDF	+++	+++	Artery and vein	++
CVVHDF	+++	+++	Large vein	++
CAVHFD	++	++++	Artery and vein	+/0
CVVHFD	++	++++	Large vein	+/0

CAVH=Continuous arteriovenous hemofiltration; CAVHD=Continuous arteriovenous hemodialysis; CAVHDF=Continuous arteriovenous hemodiafiltration; CAVHFD=Continuous arteriovenous high-flux hemodialysis; CVVH=Continuous venovenous hemofiltration; CVVHD=Continuous veno venous hemodialysis; CVVHDF=Continuous venovenous hemodiafiltration; CVVHFD=Continuous venovenous high-flux hemodialysis; SCUF=Slow continuous ultrafiltration; 0=not required; +=negligible; ++=some; +++=marked; ++++=major.

modality continues to be based on small and uncontrolled reports or small retrospective studies with inadequate group comparisons.

• It is a widespread opinion that convective treatments like high-flux hemodialysis, hemodiafiltration and hemofiltration offer a clinical advantage over standard dialysis. So far, studies have not been able to demonstrate superiority of these techniques on morbidity, mortality, and quality of life. Given the absence of evidence of superiority among the different RRT modalities, choice rests on the available equipment (membranes, pump systems), and appropriate dialysate, as well as cost and conceptual considerations.

Definitions, nomenclature

Renal replacement devices are designated as:

• "Dialyzers" working predominantly in diffusion with a countercurrent flow of blood and dialysate,

• "Hemofilters" working in convection mode.

• Newer designs permit powerful simultaneous convection and diffusion (high-flux dialysis, hemodiafiltration).

Main features of convective treatments include:

- High-flux membranes.
- High permeability to water.
- High permeability to low- and middle-molecular-weight (MW) solutes (1000–12,000 Dalton).
- High "biocompatibility."

Hemofiltration:

- Predominantly a convective technique.
- Allows removal of larger quantities of hydrophilic large MW compounds than diffusion.
- Achieves greater cytokine removal by adsorption and convection.
- Removal of inflammatory mediators has been postulated but not demonstrated to benefit patient outcome.

Hemodiafiltration:

- Performed utilizing partially hydrophilic high-flux membranes, with high sieving coefficient and reduced wall thickness. Combines diffusion and convection.
- Accurate ultrafiltration (UF) control systems make safe, large volume hemofiltration possible.
- Newer machines permit separate control of dialysate and ultrafiltration and reinfusion.
- On-line production of ultrapure dialysate and replacement fluid has made it possible to deliver safe and less costly treatments.

Convection and diffusion

- Intermittent hemodialysis equipment is only able to achieve clearance by simple diffusion.
- SLED/EDD technologies work predominantly by diffusion, although limited convection is also feasible.
- Current CRRT machines achieve solute exchanges by convection, diffusion, or both, with easier and more precise control over each component of the therapy. Blood, dialysate, and ultrafiltrate flow rates can be controlled accurately with integrated pumps, and greater dialysate or convective flows, therefore permitting, greater diffusive and convective solute clearances with CRRT, the low dialysate flow (usually 1–2 L/hour) limits diffusion, in contrast to intermittent hemodialysis, where dialysate flow can be as high as 500–800 ml/min.
- Convection-based replacement techniques (hemofiltration and hemodiafiltration) using high-flux membrane filters are aimed at maximizing the removal of so-called medium and high MW solutes (higher than 1,000 kDa up to several thousand kDa).

Kinetic considerations relevant to the present discussion are extensively reviewed in Cerda and Ronco, 2009 (see suggested readings).

Comparison among different renal replacement modalities

- CRRT techniques offer better long-term clearance of small and middle molecules than IHD or SLED. Both CRRT and SLED allow effective azotemic control, whereas IHD creates pronounced concentration peaks and poor time-averaged azotemia. Differences between modalities are more pronounced in the middle-molecule range of solutes, with superior middle-molecule clearance with CVVH compared with SLED or IHD. The superior middle and large molecule removal for CVVH is due to a combination of convection and continuous operation. While on CRRT, middle-sized solutes achieve steady state after a few days, using SLED or IHD, their plasma concentration actually increases steadily, thus reflecting the inability of the latter modalities to clear large and middle-MW toxins.

- The importance of the clearance of larger compounds is suggested by treatment trials correlating convective dose (i.e., ultrafiltration rate) with survival. Large molecular clearance may have contributed substantially to the salutary effect of higher doses in these therapies. More recent studies have shown that the addition of diffusion to convective clearance result in further improvement in patient outcome. In spite of these suggestive findings, there is no firm evidence that enhanced removal of mid- or high-MW patients leads to better patient outcomes. At the slow flow rates normally utilized in CRRT, there is no interaction between diffusive and convective clearances.

Recent randomized controlled trials on the effects of dose of RRT

Recent multicenter randomized controlled trials (RCTs) suggest CRRT is accepted as the standard of care for critically ill AKI patients with hemodynamic instability, as reflected in the design and results of the Acute Renal Failure Trial Network (ATN) Trial and the RENAL trials.

The ATN study was designed to evaluate the effects of dose on survival and renal functional recovery, based on the following premises:

- The "dose" of dialysis is a small-solute clearance-related parameter.

- Studies were not designed to determine which toxin class clearance led to better survival.

- None of these studies addresses fluid management as a "dose" variable, a consideration increasingly recognized as a critical determinant of patient outcomes (see below).

The RENAL and ATN studies suggest that a dose of 20–25 ml/kg/hour is the minimum dose to be delivered. As opposed to previous results, higher doses have not been demonstrated to improve patient outcomes, as also shown in recent meta-analysis.

There is a dose response between dialysis dose and survival. The inflexion point of the curve (Figure 10.2), beyond which further increases in dose have no additional benefit, has not been established. Therapeutic nihilism must be

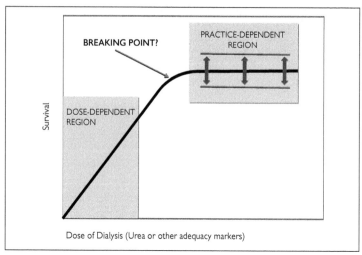

Figure 10.2 Renal replacement dose/response relationship in AKI.
Modified from Ronco C, Cruz D, Oudemans van Straaten H, et al. Dialysis dose in AKI: no time for therapeutic nihilism—a critical appraisal of the Acute Renal Failure Trial Network study. *Crit Care.* 2008;12:308.

avoided; clinicians should ensure that the dose prescribed is actually delivered. Extensive data has shown that the prescribed dose achieved in superbly designed studies such as the ATN and RENAL are rarely reproduced in common clinical practice.

The different RRT modalities utilized in these studies may have had a significant impact on patient outcomes. In the RENAL Trial performed in Australia and New Zealand, CRRT was the standard of care for critically ill AKI patients and the only therapy used in the ICU setting for more than 90 percent of patients requiring renal support. Although the baseline illness severity of the ATN and RENAL populations was similar, survival rate and rate of renal recovery were greater in the RENAL Study: All-cause mortality in the RENAL Study at *90 days* was only 45 percent (versus 53 percent at *60 days* in ATN) whereas renal recovery at 90 days among survivors was 93 percent (versus approximately 75 percent at 60 days in ATN) (Table 10.5).

Moreover, as shown in Table 10.5, both the number of required days of renal support (mean of 7.4 days and 13.1 days in the RENAL and ATN Trials, respectively) and hospital length of stay (mean of 25.2 days and 48 days in the RENAL and ATN Trials, respectively) were effectively reduced by 50 percent in the RENAL Study. Although it is not possible at this point to perform a rigorous statistical comparison of these parameters, these differences clearly have clinical relevance.

Table 10.6 Comparison of RENAL and VA/NIH studies

Variable	RENAL	VA/NIH
Mortality day 90	44.7 percent	
Mortality day 60		52.5 percent
RRT days (at 28 days)	7.4	13.1
Hospital LOS (days)	25.2	48
Dialysis dependence at day 28	13.3 percent	45.2 percent
Dialysis dependence at day 60		24.6 percent
Dialysis dependence at day 90	5.6 percent	

The RENAL study results, which are substantially better than outcomes reported historically for this patient population, warrants a critical reappraisal of the wisdom of using intermittent modalities in the management of critically ill AKI patients and further validates CRRT as the preferred technique for renal support in critically ill AKI patients.

Nutrition and outcome

Better management of volume and body fluid composition is easily achieved with CRRT. Given the importance of nutrition on the outcome of critically ill patients with AKI, CRRT could offer a theoretical advantage over IHD in this setting.

Hemodynamic stability

Older and very recent studies have consistently shown that the main advantage of continuous modalities is greater hemodynamic stability. In the ATN study, although hemodynamically "stable" patients were allocated to IHD, hypotension occurred more frequently among patients treated with IHD than CRRT and may have had an impact on their lower rate of recovery of renal function.

CRRT is associated with better tolerance to fluid removal primarily because it permits the maintenance of stable intravascular volume. In part, this is achieved by much slower fluid removal (over days rather than hours).

- Intravascular compartment volume is the main determinant of hemodynamic instability during RRT.
  - This volume results from the balance between convective removal of fluid (ultrafiltration) from plasma and fluid replenishment from the interstitium.
  - Whenever UF rate exceeds the rate of interstitium-to-plasma flow (refilling), the patient will experience hypovolemia and hemodynamic instability.
- In IHD (Figure 10.3A), rapid diffusion of urea creates a plasma-to-interstitium and interstitium-to-cell osmotic gradient that drives water to the interstitium

and to the intracellular compartment; thus, plasma volume decreases and cell edema (including neuronal edema) occurs.

• With CRRT (Figure 10.3B), the slower rate of urea clearance allows for equalization of urea concentrations between compartments and, therefore, reduces water shifts and cell edema.

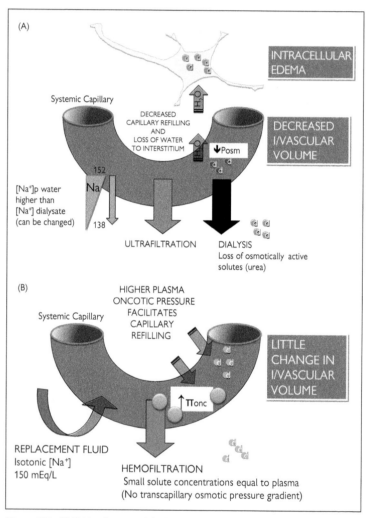

Figure 10.3 (A) Fluid and osmotic shifts during diffusive hemodialysis and (B) Fluid and osmotic shifts during convective hemofiltration.

- This is particularly important in patients with intracranial hypertension, such as head trauma and severe liver failure .
- A decrease in core temperature and peripheral vasoconstriction has been shown to decrease hypotensive episodes and may play a role in hemodynamic stability.
- With either pre- or postdilution hemofiltration, the magnitude of sodium removal is less than the amount of sodium removed with hemodialysis. This factor may contribute to better cardiovascular stability in hemofiltration.
- Although hypovolemia is the first step in dialysis-related hypotension, arterial pressure response to hypovolemia is the result of a complex interplay between decreased venous vessel capacity to sustain cardiac filling; increased arterial vascular resistances to ensure organ perfusion; and increased myocardial contractility and heart rate to maintain cardiac stroke volume. Any factor interfering with one or more of these compensatory mechanisms fosters cardiovascular instability. It is possible that convective removal of inflammatory mediators could contribute to hemodynamic stability, especially in the early phases of septic shock.

When IHD is the only modality available, the following maneuvers may help maintain stable hemodynamics:

- Change in dialysate sodium concentration: considering Gibbs-Donnan equilibrium across the dialysis membrane, to avoid the decrease in plasma osmolality caused by urea diffusion, dialysate sodium bath can be adjusted in a gradually decreasing fashion, that is, between 148 and 140 meq/l. Avoid this technique in hyponatremic patients.
- Change in ultrafiltration profile: discontinuous UF may improve refilling and avoid acute hypovolemia.
- Change in bath temperature: induction of peripheral vasoconstriction and increased sympathetic tone contributes to maintain systolic volume and peripheral resistance.
- Use of biocompatible membranes induces lesser production of inflammatory mediators increasing capillary permeability and depressing the myocardium.

Fluid overload has been shown to be a significant risk factor among critically ill patients. Recent pediatric and adult studies have established an association between fluid overload and mortality. Patients with more than10 percent fluid overload show less survival than patients without fluid overload, and patients achieving negative fluid balance have substantially lower 60-day mortality. Importantly, although use of IHD is associated with fluid gain, CRRT often permits effective volume control, in spite of their greater hemodynamic instability (Figure 10.4). Persistent fluid overload has been associated with poorer renal functional recovery.

These studies should alert the clinical community that, rather than being an innocuous process without clinical consequences, fluid overload constitutes a potentially "toxic" phenomenon that independently influences patient outcome.

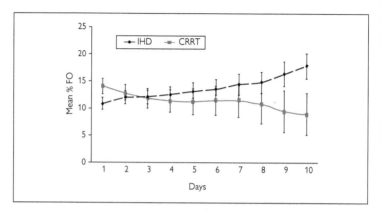

Figure 10.4 Fluid balance in patients treated with IHD and CRRT.
Modified from Bouchard J, Soroko SB, Chertow GM, Himmelfarb J, Ikizler TA, Paganini EP,
Mehta RL. Fluid accumulation, survival and recovery of kidney function in critically ill patients
with acute kidney injury.*Kidney Int.* 2009;76:422–427.
FO: Fluid overload as percent of initial weight; IHD: Intermittent hemodialysis; CRRT:
Continuous renal replacement therapy. Days: Days from admission.

Additional prospective studies are necessary to further clarify the relationship
between fluid overload and outcomes in critically ill AKI patients.

Hemofiltration of large molecules and hemadsorption

- Middle molecules:
  - Consist primarily of peptides and small proteins with MW in the range of
    1000 to 600,000 Daltons.
  - Accumulate in renal failure and contribute to the uremic toxic state.
  - Beta-2 microglobulin, with a molecular weight of 11,000 Dalton is consid-
    ered representative of these middle molecules.
  - These molecules are poorly cleared by low-flux dialysis.
  - High-flux dialysis will clear middle molecules partly by internal filtra-
    tion (convection); the convective component of high-flux dialysis can be
    enhanced in a predictable way by hemodiafiltration.

  In the last decade, it has been postulated that high-convective-dose therapies
improve the management of sepsis.

- Severe sepsis and septic shock are the primary causes of multiple organ dysfunction syndrome (MODS), the most frequent cause of death in intensive
  care unit patients.
- Many water-soluble mediators with pro- and anti-inflammatory action such as
  TNF, IL-6, IL-8, and IL-10 play a strategic role in septic syndrome.
- In intensive care medicine, blocking any one mediator has not led to a measurable outcome improvement in patients with sepsis.

- CRRT is a continuously acting therapy, which removes, in a nonselective way, pro- and anti-inflammatory mediators. The *"peak concentration hypothesis"* is the concept that cutting peaks of soluble mediators through continuous hemofiltration may help restore homeostasis.

This latter development proposes to use increased volume exchanges in hemofiltration or the combined use of adsorbent techniques.

- High-volume hemofiltration (HVHF):
  - A variant of CVVH that requires higher surface area hemofilters and ultra-filtration volumes of 35 to 80 ml/kg/h.
  - Provides higher clearance for middle/high molecular weight solutes than simple diffusive transport (CVVHD) or convection-based transport at lower volumes (CVVH).
  - Associated with practical difficulties including machinery, replacement fluid availability and cost, and accurate monitoring systems to maintain safety.
  - Studies utilizing this technique have shown preliminary evidence of benefit, but none of the studies are randomized trials of adequate statistical power to demonstrate effect conclusively.
  - Alternative technologies have utilized high cut-off hemofilters with increased effective pore size.
  - Drawbacks of such porous membranes include the loss of essential proteins such as albumin.
- Plasma filtration coupled with adsorption (CPFA) has been recently utilized in septic patients.
  - In CPFA, plasma is separated from blood and the plasma is circulated through a sorbent bed; blood is subsequently reconstituted and dialyzed with stand-ard techniques, thus achieving normalization of body-fluid composition and increased removal of protein-bound solutes and high-MW toxins.
- Recently, evidence has been obtained showing that very high volume hemofiltration applied in pulses may improve the hemodynamic stability of septic patients in septic shock, but it failed to show consistently improved survival.

Larger multicentric evidence will be necessary before such techniques are widely implemented. If benefit is demonstrated, the use of very high volume hemofiltration will require special equipment and very capable nursing able to manage such large volumes (i.e., up to 5–6 liters/hr) of ultrapure replacement fluid without error.

- Endotoxin, one of the main components of the outer membrane of gram-nega-tive bacteria, is a crucial mediator in the induction of the sepsis syndrome. Animal and human models of the syndrome demonstrate endotoxin mediated multiple organ injury, including altered hemodynamics, lung dysfunction, and AKI.

Although high levels of endotoxemia are associated with worse clinical out-comes, endotoxin-targeted treatment is controversial. Theoretically, endotoxin removal could lead to mitigation of the early septic cascade and lessening of organ injury and better survival.

Polymyxin B, an antibiotic with significant neuro and nephrotoxicity precluding its systemic use, has high affinity for endotoxin. Recently, Polymyxin B has been bound and immobilized on the surface of polystrene membrane fibers in a hemoperfusion device. Early studies suggest benefit when these devices are used in patients with septic shock and AKI; larger studies are necessary to confirm these promising results.

Suggested readings

Bellomo R, Cass A, Cole L, et al. Intensity of continuous renal-replacement therapy in critically ill patients. *N Engl J Med.* 2009;361:1627–1638.

Cerda J, Lameire N, Eggers P, et al. Epidemiology of acute kidney injury. *Clin J Am Soc Nephrol.* 2008;3:881–886.

Cerda J, Ronco C. Modalities of continuous renal replacement therapy: technical and clinical considerations. *Semin Dial.* 2009;22:114–122.

Cerda J, Sheinfeld G, Ronco C. Fluid overload in critically ill patients with acute kidney injury. *Blood Purification.* 2010;29:11–18.

Clark WR, Ronco C. Continuous renal replacement techniques. *Contrib Nephrol.* 2004;144:264–277.

Cruz D, Bellomo R, Kellum JA, de Cal M, Ronco C. The future of extracorporeal support. *Crit Care Med.* 2008;36:S243–S252.

Gibney N, Cerda J, Davenport A, et al. Volume management by renal replacement therapy in acute kidney injury. *Int J Artif Organs.* 2008;31:145–155.

KDIGO AKI Work Group: KDIGO Clinical Practice Guideline for Acute Kidney Injury. *Kidney Int.* Suppl 2012;2(1):1–138.

Palevsky PM, Bunchman T, Tetta C. The Acute Dialysis Quality Initiative—part V: operational characteristics of CRRT. *Adv Ren Replace Ther.* 2002;9:268–272.

Palevsky PM, Zhang JH, O'Connor TZ, et al. Intensity of renal support in critically ill patients with acute kidney injury. *N Engl J Med.* 2008;359:7–20.

Uchino S, Bellomo R, Kellum JA, et al. Patient and kidney survival by dialysis modality in critically ill patients with acute kidney injury. *Int J Artif Organs.* 2007;30:281–292.

Uchino S, Bellomo R, Morimatsu H, et al. Continuous renal replacement therapy: a worldwide practice survey. The beginning and ending supportive therapy for the kidney (B.E.S.T. kidney) investigators. *Intensive Care Med.* 2007;33:1563–1570.

Chapter 11

Combined kidney-lung failure

Kai Singbartl

Background

Acute kidney injury (AKI) and acute lung injury (ALI) represent serious, complex clinical problems.

AKI has traditionally been described as the abrupt loss of kidney function resulting in retention of waste products as well as dysregulation of fluid and electrolyte homeostasis. The recent introduction of two classification systems has allowed for more standardized, precise definition and staging of AKI. Both the acute kidney injury network (AKIN) classification and the "risk, injury, failure, loss" (RIFLE) classification only consider urine output and changes in serum creatinine for classification/staging.

Approximately 67 percent of all critically ill patients develop AKI. About 75 percent of patients with severe AKI require renal replacement therapy (RRT). Patients who require RRT have a hospital mortality rate of 60 percent, and only less than half of these patients recover renal function.

Acute lung injury (ALI) and its more severe form, acute respiratory distress syndrome (ARDS), are defined as:

- Bilateral pulmonary infiltrates on chest x-ray.
- Pulmonary capillary wedge pressure < 18 mmHg.
- P_aO_2/F_iO_2 <300 mmHg = ALI.
- P_aO_2/F_iO_2 <200 mmHg = ARDS.

Acute lung injury occurs with an age-adjusted incidence of 86 per 100,000 person-years and carries an in-hospital mortality rate of up to 38 percent.

The combined occurrence of AKI and ALI drastically decreases survival. The development of AKI in the setting of ALI carries an in-hospital mortality rate of 58 percent, providing strong evidence for clinically relevant kidney-lung interactions in the critically ill patient.

Various cell types, pathways, and mediators are thought to play a role in kidney-lung cross talk.

The goal of this chapter is to review the current understanding of kidney-lung-interactions.

A better understanding of this phenomenon is of utmost importance, because current clinical care is limited to supportive measures.

The effect of AKI on pulmonary function

Both human and animal studies have demonstrated that AKI can affect lung function in numerous ways (Figure 11.1). These effects go beyond those that can be expected from the typical clinical complications of AKI, such as hyperkalemia, pulmonary edema, pericarditis.

In the healthy lung, experimental AKI increases pulmonary vascular permeability and causes erythrocyte sludging in lung capillaries, interstitial edema, focal alveolar hemorrhage, and inflammatory cell infiltration. Experimental AKI also leads to down-regulation of epithelial salt and water transporters, contributing to decreased alveolar fluid clearance. It remains, however, unknown to what extent theses changes affect clinical lung function, in particular oxygenation.

To the contrary, experimental studies in the setting of combined AKI and ALI suggest that AKI exerts anti-inflammatory effects toward the lung. Acute kidney injury decreases recruitment of inflammatory cells and improves oxygenation during aseptic ALI.

The exact mechanisms of how AKI affects lung structure and function are still incompletely understood, and they are likely dependent on the underlying state of the lung. Several studies have suggested a role for leukocyte trafficking, cytokines, oxidative stress or apoptosis.

Cytokines are crucial in the initiation and progression of both AKI and ALI. AKI increases pulmonary concentrations of interleukin-6 (IL-6), interleukin-10 (IL-10), and serum amyloid 3 are increased in the healthy lung during AKI. Blockade of IL-6 or IL-10 reduces pulmonary inflammation in animal models of postischemic AKI.

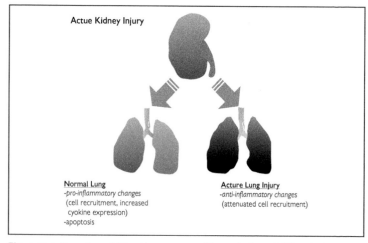

Figure 11.1 Currently available evidence suggests differential effects of AKI on the lung. Acute kidney injury has pro-inflammatory effects on the healthy lung, whereas AKI exerts anti-inflammatory effects during ALI.

Experimental data support a role for oxidative stress and its systemic effects in AKI-induced remote cellular and tissue injury. Heme oxygenase 1 is a key enzyme in the body's defense against oxidative stress, as it induces anti-inflammatory and antioxidant metabolites. Mice gene-deficient in heme oxygenase-1 show increased renal inflammation and consequently increased systemic and pulmonary IL-6 as well as increased mortality in models of postischemic AKI.

Apoptosis is a tightly regulated mechanism of cell death, during which damaged cells are removed. Numerous diseases are characterized by excessive or uncontrolled apoptosis. Enhanced apoptosis of pulmonary endothelial/epithelial cell as well as delayed apoptosis of neutrophils are hallmarks of ALI. Renal ischemia-reperfusion induces caspase-dependent apoptosis of pulmonary endothelial cells, which, in turn, effects microvascular permeability.

Leukocyte trafficking and recruitment in the context of AKI-induced lung injury remain highly controversial. Some studies have demonstrated increased recruitment of inflammatory cells, in particular neutrophils, into the healthy lung, although the effects on lung function, that is, oxygenation, remain unclear. By contrast, animal studies in models of AKI and noninfectious ALI combined have shown that AKI impairs pulmonary recruitment under these circumstances and thereby improves oxygenation. The site of the underlying mechanisms seems to be the neutrophil itself. Uremic neutrophils exhibits impaired pulmonary recruitment in both normal and uremic plasma, whereas the recruitment of normal neutrophils is not altered, either in normal or uremic plasma.

The effect of ALI on renal function

Whereas the effects of AKI on pulmonary function are still far from being understood, both clinical and experimental studies have delineated the effects of ALI on renal function and the underlying mechanisms rather well (Figure 11.2).

Hypoxemia as well as hypercarbia and acid-base disturbances resulting from ALI lead to the release of vasoactive substances, such as endothelin, angiotensin, and norepineprine. The resulting vasoconstriction decreases renal blood flow.

Many of the extrapulmonary effects of ALI are due to mechanical ventilation. Mechanical ventilation has profound effects on systemic and local hemodynamics. Mechanical ventilation can reduce venous return, pulmonary vascular resistance, and cardiac afterload and ultimately cardiac output. Mechanical ventilation also redistributes intra-renal blood flow and activates hormonal and sympathetic pathways. Functional consequences include decrease in creatinine and free water clearance as well as sodium excretion.

Beyond these direct mechanical effects, mechanical ventilation also contributes to the so-called biotrauma of the lung during ALI. Acute-lung-injury-associated biotrauma is characterized by local and systemic release of inflammatory mediators, including TNF-a, IL-1b, IL-6, and IL-8. Reduction of biotrauma by a decrease in preset tidal volumes ("lung protective" ventilation) has reduced the morbidity

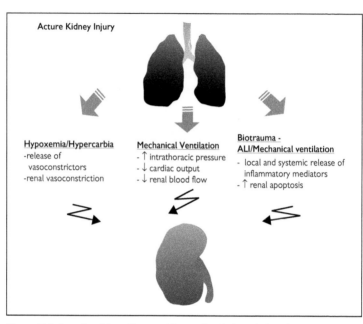

Figure 11.2 Acute lung injury affects renal function largely through three distinct mechanisms: Hypoxemia/hypercarbia lead to relaese of renal vasoconstrictors and consequently to renal hypoperfusion; mechanical ventilation increases intrathoracic pressure, subsequently decreasing venous return and cardiac output; mechanical ventilation and ALI together cause the so-called biotrauma that is characterized by local and systemic release of inflammatory mediators.

and mortality from ALI in experimental and large clinical studies and now represents a cornerstone in the management of patients with ALI.

Conclusions

Acute kidney injury remains a major clinical challenge, especially in combination with ALI.

Both clinical and experimental studies support the concept of clinically relevant kidney-lung interactions. The crosstalk between AKI and ALI is the result of both direct loss of normal organ function and inflammatory dys-regulation associated with each organ failure. Cellular as well as soluble mediators contribute to the inflammatory dysregulation in this setting.

Current clinical strategies do not offer therapeutic intervention but rather preventive or supportive measures. As for AKI, these include adequate volume control, correction of acid-base/electrolyte abnormalities, and elimination of uremic substances by renal replacement therapy. Lung protective ventilation is a centerpiece in the management of ALI. This approach minimizes both the direct mechanical effects of ventilation and the inflammatory response arising from ALI and mechanical ventilation.

Future research activities need to focus on organ cross talk, as multi-organ failure is not only the sum of loss of organ functions but also includes inflammatory dysregulation and its consequences.

Suggested readings

The Acute Respiratory Distress Syndrome Network. Ventilation with lower tidal volumes as compared with traditional tidal volumes for acute lung injury and the acute respiratory distress syndrome. *N Engl J Med.* 2000;342:1301–1308.

Grigoryev DN, Liu M, Hassoun HT, et al. The local and systemic inflammatory transcriptome after acute kidney injury. *J Am Soc Nephrol.* 2008;19:547–558.

Hassoun HT, Lie ML, Grigoryev DN, et al. Kidney ischemia-reperfusion injury induces caspase-dependent pulmonary apoptosis. *Am J Physiol Renal Physiol.* 2009; 297:F125–F137.

Hoke TS, Douglas IS, Klein CL, et al. Acute renal failure after bilateral nephrectomy is associated with cytokine-mediated pulmonary injury. *J Am Soc Nephrol.* 2007;18:155–164.

Imai Y, Parodo J, Kajikawa O, et al. Injurious mechanical ventilation and end-organ epithelial cell apoptosis and organ dysfunction in an experimental model of acute respiratory distress syndrome. *JAMA.* 2003;289:2104–2112.

Scheel PJ, Liu M, Rabb H. Uremic lung: new insights into a forgotten condition. *Kidney Int.* 2008;74:849–851.

Zarbock A, Schmolke M, Spieker T, et al. Acute uremia but not renal inflammation attenuates aseptic acute lung injury: A critical role for uremic neutrophils. *J Am Soc Nephrol.* 2006;17:3124–3131.

Chapter 12

Acute kidney injury in cirrhosis

Mitra K. Nadim and Neesh Pannu

Acute kidney injury (AKI) is a relatively frequent complication of end-stage liver disease, occurring in up to 20 percent of hospitalized patients with cirrhosis. Renal function and the development of AKI are powerful predictors of outcome in patients with cirrhosis both pre- and postorthotopic liver transplant.

Methods of assessing renal function in liver disease

Evaluation of renal function in patients with coexistent hepatic disease remains a critically important and challenging problem.
- Glomerular filtration rate (GFR) is considered the best estimate of renal function, although there is no universally accepted gold standard for measurement of GFR.
- The clearance of exogenous markers such as radiocontrast media, inulin, or radioisotopes, are considered the most accurate methods of GFR assessment, although they are not routinely used in clinical practice, for reasons of cost, convenience, and availability.
- For patients with liver disease, particularly those with advanced cirrhosis and ascites, none of the exogenous clearance markers have been rigorously studied. When properly performed, timed urinary collection of serum creatinine overcomes some of these limitations however are subject to inaccuracy due to increased tubular secretion of creatinine as GFR declines and inaccurate or incomplete urine collection.
- Estimation of GFR using mathematical equations based on serum creatinine is a simple and reliable method in the general population; however, serum creatinine remains the most commonly used clinical index of kidney function. The advantages and disadvantages of currently available methods of renal function assessment are summarized in Table 12.1.

Table 12.1 Methods of assessing renal function in liver disease

		Advantages	Disadvantages
Serum based methods	Serum creatinine	• Universally available • Inexpensive • MELD/AKI scores, current HRS definitions use this	• Affected by age, gender, muscle mass, steroids, medications • Decreased generation in liver disease • Bilirubin effect on assay • Lack of standardization of creatinine assays • Slow to rise in AKI
	Serum cystatin C	• Not affected by age, gender, muscle mass, sepsis • Simple blood test • Commercial assays are available • Appears to detect early kidney dysfunction and AKI earlier than serum creatinine	• Underestimates GFR post transplant • Dilution as with all serum markers • Variable performance of Cystatin C • Variable expense
Clearance based methods	Urinary creatinine clearance	• Inexpensive • Avoids dilution issues of serum markers	• Difficult to get accurate collections • Systematically overestimates GFR in liver disease by 10–15% especially in pts with chronic kidney disease
	Inulin	• Still considered gold standard	• Systematic plasma clearance overestimates GFR • Cumbersome
	Iothalamate	• As good as inulin in most studies	• Significant extrarenal clearance • Shown to overestimate GFR by 10–20 ml/min
	CrEDTA	• As good as inulin in most studies	• Significant extrarenal clearance • Shown to overestimate GFR by 10–20 ml/min
	DcDPTA	• As good as inulin in most studies	• Significant extrarenal clearance

Serum creatinine

- Creatinine is synthesized in the liver where it is generated by irreversible de-phosphorylation of phospho creatine, a high-energy compound.
- Daily creatinine generation varies little from day to day, but is influenced by a variety of factors including age, muscle mass, gender, and ethnicity.
- In liver cirrhosis, serum creatinine overestimates renal function for several reasons: decreased creatine production by the liver, protein calorie malnutrition, and muscle wasting. Baseline serum creatinines are consequently lower in cirrhosis than they are in the general population and a serum creatinine within the normal range does not exclude renal impairment.
- Serum creatinine values may vary widely in patients with ascites because of dilutional changes in volume status after paracentesis and with the use of diuretics. High serum bilirubin levels may affect the assays used for measurement of serum creatinine resulting in falsely low serum creatinine concentrations. Alternative methods are available; however, they are costly and not widely available. Finally variations in assay calibration among clinical laboratories may also create another source of inaccuracy.

Despite the many limitations of serum creatinine, its widespread use and access makes serum creatinne the most practical method of GFR assessment. Serum creatinine remains the basis of existing clinical definitions of AKI in patients with without renal disease and is a key component in the Model for End-Stage Liver Disease (MELD) score, which is used to prioritize patients for liver transplantation.

Creatinine based equations

The Cockcroft Gault and MDRD equations are widely used to estimate GFR in the general population, but they consistently overestimate GFR in cirrhotic patients.

- The Cockcroft Gault equation is heavily influenced by weight as a reflection of lean body mass, which is not well suited to cirrhotic patients, in whom edema and ascites may account for a large proportion of weight.
- The MDRD equation, which does not use a weight variable, may be more accurate. Several retrospective evaluations of serum creatinine based GFR estimation equations among liver transplant recipients suggest that the MDRD equations were best able to estimate GFR in comparison to radionuclotide GR assessment; however, the precision of all eGFR equations was poor and GFR estimation equations cannot be reliably used in patients with liver disease.

Ancillary testing in renal function assessment

Novel biomarkers are emerging as diagnostic tools for AKI. Only one published study has evaluated an AKI biomarker in cirrhotics to date; serum NGAL (Neutrophil Gelatinase-Associated Lipocalin) measured 2 hours after reperfusion of the liver was predictive of AKI in patients undergoing liver transplantation. Currently, two large studies are underway to assess the use of AKI biomarkers in patients with chronic liver disease in the United Kingdom. The broader study of AKI biomarkers in patients pre- and post-liver transplantation is warranted.

A variety of other investigations should also be considered in a comprehensive evaluation of renal function in this clinical setting:

• Noninvasive tests such as volumetric analysis.
• Diagnostic Doppler ultrasound.
• Urinalysis (i.e. cast scoring).
• Urine volume based on current AKI stratification criteria (RIFLE, AKIN).
• Serological analysis for hepatorenal diseases. The use of more invasive testing, such as renal biopsy should also be considered with due diligence given the potential complication possibilities present in patients with underlying hepatic diseases.

Acute kidney injury in patients with liver disease

In 2004, the Acute Dialysis Quality Initiative (ADQI) Workgroup developed a consensus definition and classification for AKI known as the RIFLE criteria, The Acute Kidney Injury Network (AKIN), an independent collaborative network consisting of experts from ADQI and several nephrology and intensive-care medicine societies, proposed to broaden the definition of AKI to include an absolute increase in serum creatinine of ≥ 0.3 mg/dL (26 μmol/L) when documented to occur within 48 hours. Once AKI is established, a staging system then defines its severity (Table 12.2). By early 2010, the RIFLE criteria has been validated in over 500,000 patients of AKI and has been shown to predict clinical outcomes with a progressive increase in mortality with worsening RIFLE class. In critically ill patients with cirrhosis, using RIFLE criteria for AKI was shown to be a good predictor of hospital survival.

Table 12.2 Definition and classification of AKI (modified RIFLE criteria)

AKI stage	Serum creatinine criteria	Urine output criteria
1 (Risk)	Increase serum creatinine of ≥ 0.3 mg/dL (≥ 26.4 μmol/L) within 48 hrs or an increase of ≥ 150–200% (1.5 to 2-fold) from baseline	<0.5 ml/kg/hour for >6 hours
2 (Injury)	Increase serum creatinine to 200–299% (> 2 to 3-fold) from baseline	<0.5 ml/kg/hour for >12 hours
3 (Failure)	Increase serum creatinine to ≥ 300% (> threefold) from baseline or serum creatinine of ≥ 4.0 mg/dL (≥ 354 μmol/L) with an acute increase of ≥ 0.5 mg/dL (44 μmol/L) or initiation of RRT	< 0.3 ml/kg/hour for 24 hours or anuria for 12 hours

Traditionally, three types of AKI have been identified

1. **Prerenal azotemia** resulting from renal hypoperfusion.
2. **Intrinsic renal failure**, most commonly acute tubular necrosis as a result of a toxic or ischemic renal insult, or interstitial nephritis.
3. **Post renal failure** resulting from urinary obstruction.
4. Patients with liver cirrhosis can develop all three kinds of AKI in addition to which they are uniquely vulnerable to a fourth type of kidney injury called hepatorenal syndrome (HRS). Hepatorenal syndrome is generally defined as functional renal failure in the setting of liver cirrhosis, which is not associated with structural damage to the kidneys but is unresponsive to fluid expansion.

Frequency

- The most common cause of AKI in hospitalized cirrhotics is prerenal AKI, accounting for approximately 68 percent of the cases. Acute kidney injury is mostly secondary to infection, hypovolemia (gastrointestinal hemorrhage, aggressive diuresis, or diarrhea), use of vasodilators, and other factors that cause renal vasoconstriction such as nonsteroidal anti-inflammatory drugs or intravenous contrast agents.
- HRS constitutes approximately 17 percent of cases of AKI in hospitalized patients with cirrhosis and up to 40 percent of patients with cirrhosis over a five-year period.

Hepatorenal Syndrome

Diagnosis

In 1996, the International Ascites Club (IAC) defined HRS as a syndrome that

- Occurs in patients with cirrhosis, portal hypertension, and advanced liver failure.
- Is characterized by impaired renal function and marked abnormalities in the arterial circulation and activity of endogenous vasoactive systems.
- Is a diagnosis of exclusion, when all other causes of renal failure have been excluded. The criteria for diagnosis of HRS are described in Table 12.3.
- The IAC further subdivided HRS into type 1 and type 2.
  - Type 1 HRS is characterized by a rapid decline in renal function defined as a doubling of serum creatinine to a level > 2.5 mg/dL or >50 percent reduction in creatinine clearance to less than 20 ml/min within two weeks. The patients are usually very sick, with marked jaundice and severe coagulopathy.
  - In type 2 HRS, renal function deteriorates more slowly with the serum creatinine increasing to greater than > 1.5 mg/dL or a CrCl decreasing to less than 40 mL/min over the course of weeks to months. The clinical presentation is that of gradual renal failure in a patient with cirrhosis and refractory ascites.

Table 12.3 International Ascites Club (IAC) definition and diagnostic criteria for hepatorenal syndrome
1. Cirrhosis with ascites
2. Serum creatinine > 1.5 mg/dL (133 µmol/L)
3. No improvement of serum creatinine (decrease to a level of < 1.5 mg/dL) following at least 2 days of diuretic withdrawal and volume expansion with albumin at 1 g/kg/day (up to a maximum of 100 g/day)
4. Absence of shock
5. No current or recent treatment with nephrotoxic drugs
6. Absence of parenchymal kidney disease as indicated by proteinuria > 500 mg/day, microhematuria (> 50 RBC per high power field) or abnormal renal ultrasonography

Pathogenesis

The pathophysiology of HRS is complex and multifactorial. The four main factors involved in the pathogenesis of HRS are:

1. Development of splanchnic vasodilation, which leads to a reduction in effective arterial blood volume and mean arterial pressure.
2. Activation of the renin-angiotensin-aldosterone system and sympathetic nervous system. This results in renal vasoconstriction and a shift in the renal autoregulatory curve to the right.
3. Development of cirrhotic cardiomyopathy. This leads to impairment of cardiac function and a relative impairment of the compensatory increase in cardiac output due to vasodilation
4. Increase in vasoactive mediators, which affect renal blood flow.

Approach to the patient with cirrhosis and AKI

- Based on the ADQI classification for AKI, AKI is defined as >1.5-fold increase in serum creatinine from baseline. However, currently, it is unknown at what level of creatinine AKI should be defined in patients with cirrhosis.
- In patients with a history of shock (septic or hypovolemic) or recent history of nephrotoxic agents, the most likely cause is ATN.
- In all others, the initial step is to discontinue diuretics or lactulose (if the patient has a history of recent diarrhea) and volume expand the patient with albumin at a dose of 1 g/kg. If there is improvement in the serum creatinine, then the most likely cause of AKI was prerenal azotemia. If there is no improvement in the serum creatinine, then the differential diagnosis includes HRS or ATN. Patients with HRS can be treated with vasoconstrictors as discussed earlier.

Differentiation of the causes of AKI can be difficult in patients with cirrhosis.

- The cause of AKI is generally distinguished by the preceding history as well as urinalysis and response to a volume challenge as described by the HRS criteria.
- Classically, prerenal AKI and HRS are described as sodium avid states with low (<10 mEq/L) urinary sodium (U_{Na}), fractional excretion of sodium (Fe_{Na}) < 1 percent, low (< 35 percent) fractional excretion of urea (Fe_{Urea}), high (> 500 mOsm/kg) urinary osmolality and a "bland" urine sediment.
- In contrast, patients with ATN frequently have a high (> 40 mEq/L) U_{Na}, high Fe_{Na} > 2 percent, high Fe_{Urea} >40 percent, a low urine osmolality (< 350 mOsm/kg) and the presences of granular casts on urine sediment.

Differentiating between prerenal and HRS may also be difficult. Prerenal AKI typically improves with volume expansion; however, with cirrhosis, assessment of intravascular volume deficit in patients who are total body sodium overloaded is difficult and may require central venous pressure to assist in management.

Treatment of patients with acute kidney injury

Treatment of AKI in cirrhosis is based on the etiology.

- In patients with prerenal AKI, treatment includes volume repletion and discontinuation of the precipitant, which is typically diuretics.
- ATN should be treated with supportive care including renal replacement therapy (RRT) if needed.
- The treatment of HRS can be broken down as in the following sections.

Pharmacologic

The mainstay of pharmacologic management of patients with HRS is the use of vasoconstrictors in order to reverse the splanchnic vasodilation (Table 12.4). Intravenous albumin therapy co-administration appears to enhance their benefit.

Table 12.4 Vasoconstrictor drugs for the treatment of hepatorenal syndrome

Drug	Dose
Terlipressin	0.5–2.0 mg intravenously every 4–6 hours
Vasopressin	0.01–0.08 U/min (continuous infusion)
Noradrenaline	0.5–3.0 mg/h (continuous infusion)
Octreotide + Midodrine	Octreotide: 100–200 µg subcutaneously three times a day Midodrine: 7.5–12.5 mg orally three times a day

- Terlipressin is a distinctive vasopressin analogue with preferential effects on the V1 receptor. Although not currently commercially available in the United States, it is the most widely used agent for type 1 HRS.
  - The doses of terlipressin used ranged from 2–12mg daily in divided doses in combination with albumin (loading dose of 1/kg up to a maximum of 100 g followed by 20–40 g/day).
  - The duration of terlipressin therapy is usually up to two weeks, with step-wise dose increments every few days, if there is no improvement in serum creatinine and no adverse effects.
  - For patients in whom there is a partial response (serum creatinine improves, but does not decrease below 1.5 mg/dL) or, in those patients who exhibit no improvement of renal function (no reduction of serum creatinine), continued treatment should be avoided.
- Vasopressin is an endogenous human hormone, which exerts its action through three vasopressin receptors: V1, V2, and V3.
  - Activation of the V1 receptor leads to vasoconstriction by vascular smooth muscle contraction. There is limited data on the efficacy of vasopressin in HRS compared to the newer analogues, particularly terlipressin. However vasopressin is widely available whereas terlipressin availability remains limited.
- Norepinephrine is a catecholamine, but its alpha-adrenergic activity makes it a potent vasoconstrictor of both the venous and arterial vasculature. Small studies have shown that in patients with type 1 HRS, norepinephrine has similar efficacy to terlipressin.
- Midodrine has the advantage of oral administration and works as an alpha-adrenergic receptor agonist causing vascular smooth muscle vasoconstriction.
- Octreotide is a somatostatin analogue used to reduce portal hypertension after variceal hemorrhage and may cause splanchnic vasoconstriction by inhibition of endogenous vasodilators such as glucagon. The combination of midodrine 7.5–12.5 mg orally and octreotide 100–200 micrograms subcutaneous, both 3 times daily, together with 10–20g of intravenous albumin daily has been shown to improve GFR in patients with HRS type 1.

Transjugular intrahepatic portosystemic shunt (TIPS)

- TIPS improves refractory ascites and minimizes the complication of hepatic encephalopathy in those with Child-Pugh Score (CPS) less than 11 and minimal signs of encephalopathy.
- It should be considered in patients with refractory ascites requiring frequent. TIPS may improve kidney function in 45–50 percent of those with CPS < 11.

Extracorporeal therapy

- The goal of extracorporeal support systems is to bridge liver failure patients to either transplantation or functional recovery, by means of detoxification,

assistance with biosynthesis of key metabolic products, and regulation of inflammation.
- Although a number of extracorporeal support devices have been tested for the management of HRS, most of the studies are small and uncontrolled.
- Extracorporeal albumin-containing dialysate such as Molecular Adsorbent Recirculation System (MARS) and Single Pass Albumin Dialysis, are considered experimental therapy, and their use is currently not recommended outside clinical investigation.

Renal replacement therapy (RRT)

- Renal replacement therapy improves short-term survival in patients with severe AKI and, therefore, should be regarded as supportive therapy in patients with cirrhosis and AKI only when the classic indications for dialysis are present (i.e., volume overload, azotemia, hyperkalemia, metabolic acidosis) among patients who are otherwise deemed to have a reversible decompensation of their liver disease or are liver-transplant candidates.
- With regard to modality of renal replacement therapy, continuous renal replacement therapy (CRRT) use may be advantageous in the management of HRS patients with AKI who are hemodynamically unstable or at risk of elevated intracranial pressure causing or complicating hepatic encephalopathy.

Liver transplantation

The definitive therapy for HRS is liver transplantation.

- As the waiting time for liver transplantation has increased, the incidence of pretransplant renal dysfunction and RRT has also increased. However, the level of renal dysfunction and the duration of renal dysfunction (including RRT) beyond which renal recovery is not possible after liver transplant are unknown.
- Currently there are no standard criteria for the evaluation, selection, and/or allocation of a kidney with a liver transplant. For those at risk for nonrecovery of renal function, combined liver-kidney transplantation may be justified. (Table 12.5).

Table 12.5 Recommendations for combined liver-kidney transplantation

1. Patients with end-stage renal disease
2. Patients with chronic kidney disease with GFR $\leq$ 30 ml/min
3. Patients with acute kidney injury/HRS with creatinine $\geq$ 2 mg/dL or dialysis $\geq$ 8 weeks
4. Patients with evidence of chronic kidney disease and kidney biopsy demonstrating > 30% glomerulosclerosis or 30% fibrosis

Other criteria recommended are the presence of co-morbidities such as diabetes, hypertension, age > 65, other preexisting renal disease along with proteinuria, renal size and duration of elevated serum creatinine

Suggested readings

Eason JD, Gonwa TA, Davis CL, et al. Proceedings of Consensus Conference on Simultaneous Liver Kidney Transplantation (SLK). *Am J Transplant.* 2008;8:2243–2251.

Francoz C, Glotz D, Moreau R, et al. The evaluation of renal function and disease in patients with cirrhosis. *J Hepatol.* 2010;52:605–613.

Garcia-Tsao G, Parikh CR, Viola A. Acute kidney injury in cirrhosis. *Hepatology.* 2008;48:2064–2077.

Gines P, Schrier RW. Renal failure in cirrhosis. *N Engl J Med.* 2009;361:1279–1290.

Gonwa TA, Jennings L, Mai ML, et al. Estimation of glomerular filtration rates before and after orthotopic liver transplantation: evaluation of current equations. *Liver Transpl.* 2004;10:301–309.

Jenq CC, Tsai MH, Tian YC, et al. RIFLE classification can predict short-term prognosis in critically ill cirrhotic patients. *Intensive Care Med.* 2007;33:1921–1930.

MacAulay J, Thompson K, Kiberd BA, et al. Serum creatinine in patients with advanced liver disease is of limited value for identification of moderate renal dysfunction: are the equations for estimating renal function better? *Can J Gastroenterol.* 2006;20:521–526.

Ricci Z, Cruz D, Ronco C. The RIFLE criteria and mortality in acute kidney injury: A systematic review. *Kidney Int.* 2008;73:538–546.

Sagi SV, Mittal S, Kasturi KS, et al. Terlipressin therapy for reversal of type 1 hepatorenal syndrome: a meta-analysis of randomized controlled trials. *J Gastroenterol Hepatol.* 2010;25:880–885.

Salerno F, Gerbes A, Gines P, Wong F, Arroyo V. Diagnosis, prevention and treatment of hepatorenal syndrome in cirrhosis. *Gut.* 2007;56:1310–1318.

Chapter 13

Renal disorders in pregnancy

Arun Jeyabalan

Acute kidney disease in pregnancy poses a unique challenge since there are two patients: the mother and her fetus. In addition, the profound renal and cardiovascular adaptations of pregnancy impact diagnosis and management. A multidisciplinary team approach including critical care specialists, maternal-fetal medicine specialists/high risk obstetricians, nephrologists, and neonatologists is essential due to complex decision-making that is often necessary.

Definitions

Acute kidney injury (AKI) occurring during pregnancy, labor, delivery, and/or the pospartum period is referred to as pregnancy-related AKI (PR-AKI). Two major categories of PR-AKI are:

1. diagnoses that are specific and unique to pregnancy
2. other causes that happen to coincide with pregnancy.

Specific diagnostic criteria for acute renal failure, even in the nonpregnant population, are often vague and variable, thus confounding the medical litera-ture and affecting evidence based care. In an effort to standardize the definition, the AKI Network, a multidisciplinary group, defines AKI as an abrupt (within 48 hours) reduction in kidney function defined as an absolute increase in serum creatinine of ≥ 0.3 mg/dL, a percentage increase in serum creatinine of ≥ 50 percent (1.5-fold from baseline), or a reduction in urine output (documented oliguria of <0.5 ml/kg per hour for more than six hours) (see chapter 1). With pregnancy, understanding the normal physiologic changes in the renal and car-diovascular systems is fundamental to proper diagnosis and management.

Renal adaptations during pregnancy

Anatomic and physiologic changes occur as early as the first trimester.

1. Anatomic changes:
   a. Size and volume of the kidneys increase due to the increase in blood volume and capacity of the collecting system.

b. Dilation of the collecting system with hydronephrosis and hydroureter occurs in 80 percent of women by midpregnancy, likely secondary to hormonal effects resulting in smooth muscle relaxation. Right-sided ureteral dilation is greater than the left because of compression by the enlarged and dextro-rotated uterus as well as the ovarian vascular plexus at the level of the pelvic brim.

2. Physiologic changes:

a. Increase in renal blood flow and glomerular filtration rate (GFR) is one of the earliest and dramatic changes in pregnancy. This is associated with a marked reduction of systemic vascular resistance as well as an increase in cardiac output and plasma volume. Progesterone, relaxin, and other pregnancy hormones are likely responsible for these hemodynamic changes. By the third trimester, renal plasma flow is 50–85 percent above nonpregnant levels with a slight decline toward the very end of gestation. Secondarily, GFR also increases by 40–65 percent. These changes affect the normal ranges for standard laboratory parameters and have practical implications for the care of the pregnant woman (Table 13.1). For example, a serum creatinine of 0.9 mg/dL considered to be normal for an adult would be abnormal in a healthy pregnant woman. The increased GFR also results in an increase in urinary protein excretion and often glucosuria.

b. Volume and sodium balance. Despite the increase in GFR, there is a net sodium retention of 900–950 mEq due to tubular reabsorption and total-body water increases by 6–8 liters over the course of pregnancy

Table 13.1 Normal Ranges for laboratory parameters in pregnancy

Variable	Direction of change compared to nonpregnant values	Approximate normal value in pregnancy
Serum creatinine	↓	0.5 mg/dl
Blood urea nitrogen (BUN)	↓	9.0 mg/dl
Uric acid	↓	2.0–3.0 mg/dl
pCO_2	↓	27–32 mmHg
pH	↑	7.40–7.45
Serum bicarbonate	↓	18–20 mEq/L
Creatinine clearance	↑	↑ ~25% above baseline
Urinary protein excretion	Variable to ↑	Up to 300 mg/24 hours
Urinary glucose excretion	Variable to ↑	Variable

c. Acid-base homeostasis. The increased minute ventilation of pregnancy results in a respiratory alkalosis (pCO_2 is reduced by ~10mmHg). A partial compensatory metabolic acidosis occurs via increased renal bicarbonate excretion. The resulting increase in CO_2 gradient across the placenta facilitates gas exchange and is beneficial for the fetus; however, it reduces the maternal capacity to buffer acids. These physiologic acid-base changes are important in the care of the pregnant woman, particularly in the ICU setting.

General principles of evaluation

Initial evaluation of PR-AKI should consist of a detailed history, physical examination, and laboratory assessment. *The underlying cause is often obvious based on clinical history, for example, severe obstetric hemorrhage.* Assessment of hemodynamic stability is important as many of these women will require ICU management. Urine output and serum creatinine are key laboratory components in the diagnosis of AKI. Electrolytes and complete blood count are useful as these can be primarily or secondarily affected by renal failure. Urine electrolytes and microscopy can be helpful in further determining the etiology of AKI. Specialized serologic tests can also be used to investigate other causes of AKI. Renal biopsy, although an option, may be associated with higher morbidity during pregnancy. In most cases, diagnoses can be made without a biopsy and empiric treatment started. An exception may be with sudden and unexplained renal deterioration in midpregnancy where maternal therapy without iatrogenic preterm delivery may be beneficial. A multidisciplinary approach is warranted in making such decisions.

The conventional framework of prerenal, intrarenal, and postrenal to determine the cause of AKI is also useful in pregnancy.

• Prerenal AKI occurs secondary to reduced renal perfusion. Intravascular volume depletion (as with hemorrhage or dehydration), hypotension (as in septic shock), low cardiac output or combinations of these factors are common causes of prerenal PR-AKI. If not apparent based on the clinical scenario, fractional excretion of sodium and urinary sodium may be used in differentiating between prerenal and intrarenal etiologies. With prerenal causes, both would be expected to be low (fractional excretion of sodium <1 percent and urine sodium <20 mEq) since the kidney retains the ability to concentrate urine appropriately.

• Intrarenal AKI or intrinsic renal damage may occur if prerenal causes are severe, prolonged, or uncorrected resulting in acute tubular and/or cortical necrosis. Alternatively, intrarenal AKI may be caused by direct kidney injury such as with nephrotoxins (e.g., certain drugs) or immune-mediated injury (e.g., glomerulonephritis, lupus). Urine sodium and fractional excretion of sodium would be higher with intrinsic causes, >40 mEq/L and >2 percent, respectively. Lower urine osmolality with granular or cellular casts may also be observed.

- Postrenal AKI refers to downstream obstruction that can result in renal failure such as with urethral or bilateral ureteral obstruction. Ultrasound is generally used as the first line for imaging of the urinary tract during pregnancy.

General principles of management

Basic principles of PR-AKI management are:

1. Treat the underlying cause. *By far, the most common cause of PR-AKI is reduced renal perfusion.* Specific etiologies include hypovolemia related to acute blood loss such as with intra- or postpartum hemorrhage, placental abruption or placenta previa, hypotension such as with septic shock, or low cardiac output as with cardiac failure. In each situation, addressing the cause, for example, stopping ongoing hemorrhage is fundamental. Specific treatments are discussed in the following section.

2. Prevent progression of kidney damage. *The most important tenet of management with PR-AKI is maintaining adequate renal perfusion to limit ongoing damage and reverse any pre-ischemic changes.* This can be done with intravenous crystalloid or colloid fluid administration; however, with severe obstetric hemorrhage and/or disseminated intravascular coagulation, packed red blood cells and other blood products may be indicated. Clinical status, urine output, and pulmonary function can be used to guide volume resuscitation. In complex situations, invasive hemodynamic monitoring may be helpful. All nephrotoxic medications should be stopped or at least dosed appropriately to prevent further renal decline. Pharmacologic therapies for PR-AKI are secondary; vaso-active and diuretic medications should be used with caution as they may affect uterine blood flow, placental perfusion, and fetal well-being. Postrenal contributions to renal failure, such as ureteral obstruction by the pregnant uterus, may be temporized by ureteral stents or percuta-neous nephrostomy if needed.

3. Maintain supportive care. *This includes correcting hyperkalemia, metabolic acidosis, and anemia due to AKI.* Hyperkalemia may be treated with glucose/insulin and/or polystyrene sulfonate, a potassium-binding resin. Metabolic acidosis may be acutely corrected using IV bicarbonate, while the under-lying cause is being addressed. The physiologic respiratory alkalosis must be taken into account when addressing acid-base issues in the pregnant woman. Anemia should be acutely treated with red blood cell transfu-sion. Chronic anemia due to reduced erythropoiesis can be treated with exogenous erythropoietin, although higher doses are often needed dur-ing pregnancy. Renal replacement therapy (RRT, dialysis) may be needed. Indications are similar to nonpregnant patient:
   - Volume overload.
   - Hyperkalemia refractory to medical management.

- Metabolic acidosis.
- Symptomatic uremia.

Both hemodialysis and peritoneal dialysis can be used during pregnancy. Hemodialysis is generally used in the acute setting when a rapid response is needed. The precise timing and thresholds for initiating RRT for PR-AKI are not well defined. Expert recommendations include an increase in dialysis time and frequency, keeping serum urea <45–60 mg/dL, and minimizing fluid shifts and hypotension, which can adversely affect the pregnancy. With PR-AKI, dialysis is often temporary until there is recovery of renal function.

4. Optimize fetal well-being *Fetal well-being and neonatal outcomes are closely tied to maternal status.* In general, maternal health comes first; however, fetal status should be optimized whenever possible. Adequate blood flow to the uterus and placenta is a key factor in fetal well-being; therefore, severe hypotension and intravascular volume depletion should be avoided and treated promptly. Fetal monitoring is based on gestational age. For viable pregnancies (> 23–24 weeks), assessment of fetal well-being is recommended. Continuous or intermittent fetal heart rate monitoring and/ or biophysical profile assessment by ultrasound can be used, depending on the clinical situation. If delivery is indicated prior to 34 weeks, then antenatal glucocorticoids (betamethasone or dexamethasone) should be administered to reduce neonatal morbidity and mortality. Neonatologists should be involved if delivery is a consideration.

Pregnancy-specific causes and management of AKI

Hypertensive disorders of pregnancy

Preeclampsia and HELLP syndrome

Preeclampsia is a pregnancy-specific disorder that affects 5–10 percent of pregnancies. Diagnosis is based on new onset of hypertension and proteinuria during pregnancy. Multiple organs including the maternal brain, lungs, kidneys, liver, platelets, as well as placental function can be affected with severe preeclampsia. HELLP syndrome is considered a severe variant of preeclampsia. Diagnostic criteria are presented in Table 13.2. Systemic features of preeclampsia include increased peripheral vascular resistance, endothelial dysfunction, vasospasm, activation of the coagulation and inflammatory cascades, and platelet aggregation, which can ultimately lead to ischemia and multi-organ dysfunction including AKI. The precise cause of preeclampsia is not known. A hypothesized mechanism is reduced or impaired placental perfusion leading to maternal vascular dysfunction possibly via release of placental factors.

Preeclampsia and related disorders are the most common cause of PR-AKI with an incidence of 1.5–2 percent; however, the majority of women with preeclampsia do not develop AKI. Renal plasma flow and GFR are reduced by approximately 24 percent and 32 percent, respectively, with preeclampsia compared

Table 13.2 Classification of hypertensive disorders of pregnancy

Mild preeclampsia	• New onset of sustained elevated blood pressure after 20 weeks' gestation in a previously normotensive woman (≥140 mmHg systolic or ≥90 mmHg diastolic on at least two occasions 6 hours apart)
	• Proteinuria of at least 1+ on a urine dipstick or ≥300 mg in a 24 hour urine collection after 20 weeks'
Severe preeclampsia (above criteria plus any of the items listed)	• Blood pressure ≥160 mmHg systolic or ≥110 mmHg diastolic
	• Urine protein excretion of at least 5 grams in a 24-hour collection
	• Neurologic disturbances (visual changes, headache, seizures, coma)
	• Pulmonary edema
	• Hepatic dysfunction (elevated liver transaminases or epigastric pain)
	• Renal compromise (oliguria <500 cc/24 hours or elevated serum creatinine concentration ≥ 1.2 mg/dL in women with no history of renal disease)
	• Thrombocytopenia
	• Placental abruption, fetal growth restriction, or oligohydramnios (low amniotic fluid index)
Eclampsia	• Seizures in a preeclamptic women not attributed to other causes
HELLP syndrome	• Presence of hemolysis, elevated liver enzymes, and low platelets. This may or may not occur in the presence of hypertension and is often considered a variant of preeclampsia

to normal third-trimester values. Often, AKI is associated a superimposed insult such as hemorrhage or disseminated intravascular coagulation (DIC) which can lead to acute intravascular volume depletion and maternal renal failure. Acute tubular necrosis is most common with preeclampsia. Short term RRT is required in an estimated 10–50 percent of preeclampsia-associated AKI.

The only effective cure for this progressive condition is delivery of the fetus and placenta. Mode of delivery (vaginal versus c-section) is dependent on clinical and obstetric factors. Supportive care with IV fluids and administration of blood and blood products as indicated is imperative to prevent progression of AKI. Blood pressure control is important to prevent maternal cerebrovascular accidents. Intravenous magnesium sulfate is used to prevent seizures; circulating concentrations should be monitored with AKI given the risk of respiratory depression.

Acute fatty liver of pregnancy (AFLP)
Acute fatty liver of pregnancy (AFLP) is less common, occurring in 1/5,000–1/10,000 pregnancies and can result in rapid progression and hepatic failure. Nausea, vomiting, abdominal pain, and malaise are presenting features. Laboratory abnormalities include elevated liver transaminases, hyperbilirubinemia, elevated ammonia, coagulation abnormalities, hypoglycemia, low antithrombin III, and

modest elevations in creatinine. As with preeclampsia associated AKI, superimposed insults can accelerate renal decline. Treatment consists of delivery and supportive care of the mother. Liver transplantation may be required in severe cases.

Thrombotic thrombocytopenic purpura (TTP)/Hemolytic uremic syndrome (HUS)

These are not pregnancy-specific conditions, but they are briefly discussed here because, when coincident with pregnancy, TTP/HUS can present very much like severe preeclampsia, HELLP syndrome, and/or AFLP. Table 13.3 provides some general principles in differentiating between these conditions. TTP/HUS is more common in women (70 percent) and during pregnancy (13 percent) with significant long-term mortality (range of 8 to 44 percent) and morbidity.

Table 13.3 Differential diagnosis of preeclampsia, acute fatty liver of pregnancy, TTP, and HUS*

	Pregnancy-specific diagnoses		Diagnoses not unique to pregnancy	
	Preeclampsia/ HELLP syndrome	Acute fatty liver of pregnancy (AFLP)	Thrombotic thrombocytopenic purpura (TTP)	Hemolytic uremic syndrome (HUS)
Onset	Usually 3rd trimester	Close to term	Median 23 weeks	Often postpartum
Primary/ Unique Clinical Manifestation	Hypertension and proteinuria	Nausea, vomiting, malaise	Neurologic symptoms	Renal involvement
Purpura	Absent	Absent	Present	Absent
Fever	Absent	Absent	Present	Absent
Hemolysis	Mild	Mild	Severe	Severe
Platelets	Variable (normal or low)	Variable (normal or low)	Low	Variable (normal or low)
Coagulation studies	Variable	Abnormal	Normal	Normal
Hypoglycemia	Absent	Present	Absent	Absent
vWF Multimers	Absent	Absent	Present	Present
Primary treatment	Delivery	Delivery	Plasmapheresis	Plasmapheresis

*The diagnosis may be confusing. Presence or absence of above features is not absolute, but may assist in the diagnosis. Precise diagnosis can often be made only after delivery. Preeclampsia, HELLP syndrome, and acute fatty liver of pregnancy resolve soon after delivery.

AKI is estimated to occur in two-thirds of patients, with a substantial proportion developing chronic renal insufficiency and hypertension. Although delivery is the proper treatment for preeclampsia-related disorders and AFLP, timely institution of plasmapheresis is the primary therapy for TTP/HUS. Often, the precise diagnosis is not made until after delivery; preeclampsia, HELLP syndrome, and AFLP would improve with delivery, whereas TTP/HUS would not. Glucocorticoids and aspirin are also treatment considerations. Supportive therapy and a multidisciplinary team approach are of key importance in the management of these women.

Volume depletion

Blood flow to the uterus increases markedly from 50 cc/minute before pregnancy to approximately 1,000 cc/minute at full term. Thus, obstetric hemorrhage can be rapid and massive, leading to acute intravascular volume depletion and organ damage including AKI. Pregnancy-related bleeding can occur in any trimester. Common causes and management are outlined in Table 13.4. Correcting the underlying cause along with aggressive fluid resuscitation, replacement with blood and blood products, and correction of coagulation abnormalities are basic management principles with obstetric hemorrhage.

Infections

As with nonpregnant individuals, sepsis can lead to intravascular volume depletion, hypotension, and organ dysfunction including AKI. Common infections that can lead to sepsis in pregnancy are:

1. Pyelonephritis—This occurs in 1–2 percent of pregnancies and is associated with significant maternal and fetal/neonatal complications including sepsis, preterm labor, and adult respiratory distress syndrome. Many of the physiologic changes predispose pregnant women to ascending infection of the urinary tract such as ureteral dilation, stasis related to smooth muscle relaxation, pressure on the ureters and bladder by the uterus, and possible increased susceptibility to endotoxin mediated damage. E.coli is the most common organism, followed by other gastrointestinal organsisms such as Klebsiella, Proteus, and enterococcus.

2. Chorioamnionitis—refers to Intrauterine infection involving the chorion and amniotic membranes, most commonly resulting from ascending infection from the lower genital tract. Although chorioamnionitis is common, bacteremia and sepsis related to this infection are not. These infections are often polymicrobial and caused by organisms commonly found in the lower genital tract including peptostreptococcus, Gardnerella, E. coli, Group B streptococcus, and anaerobes. Antibiotic therapy alone is usually inadequate because of poor penetration of the uterine cavity and evacuation of the uterine contents is needed.

3. Septic abortion—Although uncommon in the United States after the legalization of abortion, septic abortion is associated with significant maternal morbidity including AKI and mortality worldwide. Microbial spectrum and treatment is similar to chorioamnionitis.

Table 13.4 Common causes of obstetric hemorrhage*

	Timing	Description	Managment
Ectopic pregnancy	First trimester	Pregnancy that implants outside of the uterus—fallopian tube is the most common site. Rupture of the tube is associated with severe hemorrhage.	Immediate surgical intervention to remove the pregnancy and stop bleeding is warranted if patient is actively bleeding and hemodynamically unstable. More conservative surgical options and/or medical therapies can be used if hemodynamically stable.
Induced or spontaneous abortion	First or second trimester	Persistent, heavy bleeding is often due to products of conception that are retained within the uterine cavity	Dilation of the cervix and curettage of the uterus (D&C) is generally done if heavy bleeding and/or hemodynamic compromise
Placenta previa	Second or third trimester	Implantation of the placenta over the internal os of the cervix which can result in heavy vaginal bleeding, usually painless	Delivery by cesarean section is recommended for heavy, active bleeding. Expectant management may be considered if the bleeding is self-limited or mild
Placental abruption (or abruptio placenta)	Second or third trimester	Separation of the placenta from the uterine wall before delivery of the fetus. Usually presents as vaginal bleeding and severe abdominal pain, uterine tenderness, contractions	Severe abruption with complete separation of the placenta can lead to significant maternal bleeding, coagulopathy, fetal distress and death. Treatment is stabilization of maternal status, delivery, and supportive care. Mild or partial abruptions can be managed expectantly.
Intra- or Postpartum hemorrhage	During or after delivery (usually within 48 hours)	Severe vaginal or intra-abdominal bleeding during or after delivery. Most common reason is uterine atony (failure of the uterus to contract). Other reasons include retained placenta, genital tract lacerations, coagulopathy, placenta accreta (abnormal placental implantation), rupture or inversion of the uterus	Treatment is based on cause. For uterine atony, medical and conservative surgical therapies are used to improve uterine tone; if unsuccessful and bleeding is intractable, then hysterectomy may be indicated.

*In all cases of obstetric hemorrhage, correcting the underlying cause along with aggressive fluid resuscitation, replacement with blood and blood products as indicated, and correction of coagulation abnormalities are basic principles of management.

4. Pneumonia—Antibiotic therapy along with supportive measures such as intravenous hydration, pressors, and ventilatory support as needed are the mainstays of treatment. Initial antibiotic selection should be broad spectrum with attention to local and hospital-based microbiology and susceptibilities. Directed antibiotic therapy based on microbial culture and sensitivities can follow.

Obstruction

Urinary tract obstruction, as a cause of AKI during pregnancy is uncommon. However, the over distended uterus is a particular risk factor in pregnancy. Contributing factors include:

- Polyhydramnios (increased amniotic fluid).
- Multifetal gestation (twins and more).
- Large uterine fibroids.

Ultrasound is used for initial diagnosis; CT scan and/or pyelogram can be used if further work-up is needed. Cystoscopy with retrograde ureteral stent placement or percutaneous nephrostomy can be used to relieve or bypass the obstruction. Delivery can be considered depending on gestational age and is often the definitive treatment.

Amniotic fluid embolus

Amniotic fluid embolus or "anaphylactoid syndrome of pregnancy" refers to the sudden onset of fulminant respiratory failure, hypoxemia, cardiogenic shock, hypotension, and is often accompanied by disseminated intravascular coagulation and multi-organ failure including AKI. The precise cause is unclear, although initial case series described squamous cells and mucin of fetal origin in the pulmonary vasculature. Maternal mortality is estimated to be 22 percent, with older studies reporting rates of greater than 60 percent. Quick recognition is imperative. Treatment consists of rapid resuscitation with cardiopulmonary support and correction of coagulopathy.

Other causes of AKI not specific to pregnancy

In otherwise unexplained PR-AKI, it is important to consider other causes of AKI that tend to occur in women of reproductive age and may just be coincident with pregnancy. Detailed lists of these and other chronic causes of renal failure are discussed elsewhere. Important considerations are autoimmune etiologies (lupus, glomerulonephritis, IgA nephritis) and drugs (aminoglycosides, nonsteroidal anti-inflammatory drugs). Differentiating between acute glomerulonephritis and preeclampsia may be particularly problematic in the late second and early third trimester but crucial, because treatments are different. Some distinguishing features that point toward glomerulonephritis include systemic symptoms (lupus symptoms, preceding infections), active urinary sediment (hematuria, red cell casts), nephrotic range proteinuria (>2 grams), positive ANA, autoantibodies, and abnormal complement levels. Another clinical challenge is in the woman with preexisting renal disease who becomes pregnant. Differentiating between worsening renal disease and superimposed preeclampsia is difficult and often requires close inpatient observation and multidisciplinary decision making with attention to gestational age of the fetus.

Suggested readings

Burton R, Belfort MA, Etiology and managment of hemorrhage. In Dildy GA, III et al. eds. *Critical Care Obstetrics*. Malden, MA: Blackwell; 2004:298–311.

Deering S, Seiken G, Acute renal failure. In Dildy GA, Belfort MA, eds. *Critical Care Obstetrics*, 4th edn. Malden MA: Blackwell;2004:372–379.

Gammill HS, Jeyabalan A. Acute renal failure in pregnancy. *Crit Care Med*. 2005;33(10 Suppl): S372–S384.

Gifford RW, August PA, Cunningham FG, et al. et al., Report of the National High Blood Pressure Working Group on Research on Hypertension in Pregnancy. *Am J Ob Gyn*. 2000;183:S1–S22.

Jeyabalan A, Conrad KP, *Renal physiology and pathophysiology in pregnancy*. In Schrier RW, ed. *Renal and Electrolyte Electrolyte Disorders*. Philadelphia: Lippincott Williams & Wilkins;2010: 462–518.

Lindheimer MD, Roberts JM, F.G. Cunningham FG, *Chesley's Hypertensive Disorders in Pregnancy*. 3rd ed. San Diego: Elsevier; 2009.

Mehta R, Kellum JA, Shah SVet al. Acute Kidney Injury Network: Report of an initiative to improve outcomes in acute kidney injury. *Crit Care*. 2007;11:R31.

Thadhani R, Pascual M, Bonventre J. Acute renal failure. *N Engl J Med*. 1996;334(22): 1448–1460.

Chapter 14

Renal disorders in pediatrics

Christina Nguyen and Michael L. Moritz

There are a wide variety of renal diseases in children that are rarely or may never be encountered in the adult population. Many of these conditions can be complicated by critical illnesses that would require management in the intensive care unit. This chapter will discuss the most common renal disorders in children that could present or be complicated by a critical illness.

Hemolytic uremic syndrome (HUS)

Hemolytic uremic syndrome is a clinical diagnosis describing a triad of findings: acute renal failure, microangiopathic hemolytic anemia, and thrombocytopenia. Hemolytic uremic syndrome can be classified as either diarrheal associated (D+ HUS) or nondiarrheal associated (D– HUS) also referred to as atypical HUS. The etiology and pathogenesis of each form of HUS are different, with D+ HUS occurring in over 95 percent of cases.

I. D+ HUS (Typical HUS).
    a. Pathogenesis: D+ HUS is the childhood form of HUS immediately pre-ceded by a diarrheal illness and is closely linked to the Shiga-toxin enterohemorrhagic producing *Escherichia coli* (STEC), commonly implicated in the serotype *E. coli* 0157:H7.
    b. Epidemiology: D+ HUS most often occurs in summer months, primar-ily affecting children between 1 and 5 years of age. Incidence varies by region, but is thought to be between 0.4–1.1 cases per 100,000 chil-dren under 16 years of age. The majority of patients with HUS develop some degree of renal insufficiency and two-thirds will require dialysis. The mortality of HUS is reported to be between 3 and 5 percent, and death due to HUS is nearly always associated with severe extrarenal disease.
    c. Presentation: Symptoms typically occur 3–7 days after exposure, and diarrhea becomes bloody in the majority of patients. Diarrhea begins to subside and the child begins to appear pale with decreased urine output noted. Patients can have severe colitis and brisk hemolysis can be associated with bilirubin gallstones. Elevation of pancreatic enzymes is common and overt pancreatitis can develop. Glucose intolerance

occurs in the minority of children with HUS. Central nervous system involvement is common and often presents as lethargy, irritability, or seizures. More severe cases of central nervous system disease may present with cerebral edema. Myocardial ischemia is also fortunately rare, but elevated Troponins can be appreciated.

d. Diagnosis: The diagnosis of HUS is clinical, involving the classic triad of microangiopathic hemolytic anemia, thrombocytopenia, and acute renal insufficiency. Haptoglobin levels are low and LDH is significantly elevated. Coomb's testing will be negative as this is not an autoimmune process. Schistocytes and red blood cell fragments are apparent on blood smear.

e. Treatment: Treatment of HUS is supportive. General management of acute renal failure includes appropriate fluid and electrolyte management, antihypertensive therapy, and initiation of renal replacement therapy (RRT). Judicious volume expansion followed by a continuous infusion of 0.9 percent sodium chloride normal saline is thought to be renal-protective, limiting the amount of microangiopathic damage. Antidiarrheal drugs and antimicrobial therapy should be avoided. Transfusion of packed red blood cells is needed when hemoglobin is falling rapidly or drops below 7 g/dL. Thrombocytopenia can be profound, but platelet transfusion should be limited to those who require a surgical procedure or are actively bleeding.

II. D- HUS (atypical HUS)
   a. Pathogenesis: Atypical HUS describes the clinical presentation of HUS without preceding diarrhea or vero-toxin-related illness. Almost all patients with atypical HUS have a defect in the alternative complement pathway. Mutations for complement Factor H (FH), Factor I (FI), and membrane co-factor protein (CMP) are associated with HUS. The most commonly described defect is mutation in FH gene. Factor H antibodies are reported in approximately 10 percent of case of D-HUS.
   b. Clinical presentation: Patients with aypical HUS often have the onset of disease without a previous gastrointestinal infection; however, other types of infection may precede HUS. D-HUS can have an insidious and protracted course. In cases of onset in infancy, there is likely to be marked hypocomplementemia and severe FH deficiency. When the disease is familial, individual families tend to have a distinctive pattern of presentation and outcome. Hypertension is frequent and severe. Proteinuria is common and renal function tends to fluctuate.
   c. Treatment of atypical HUS includes supportive therapy similar to D+ HUS, but also early initiation of plasma exchange. Fresh—frozen plasma contains FH at physiological concentrations. Treatment protocols are variable, but plasma-exchange should be initiated within the first three days of illness. Steroids should be avoided and anticoagulant

therapy has not been proven beneficial. Eculizumab, a complement inhibitor that blocks the activation of the terminal complement cascade, thereby preventing the generation of the proinflammatory and prothrombotic molecules C5a and C5b-9, has shown to be effective therapy in some forms of D-HUS.

Acute glomerulonephritis

I. Poststreptococcal glomerulonephritis (PSGN).
   a. Pathogenesis: Poststreptococcal glomerulonephritis is an immune complex disease induced by specific nephritogenic strains of group A beta-hemolytic streptococcus.
   b. Epidemiology: PSGN is the most common renal pathology in underdeveloped countries. In tropical areas, this is a complication of pyoderma due to infectious with beta hemolytic streptococcus. In countries with milder climate, this is often a complication of pharyngitis during the winter months. The disease has seasonal character, and in some areas epidemics occur cyclically. The male to female ratio is 2:1 and is most common in children aged 3–12 years. The risk of developing PSGN after an infection with nephrogenic strain of GABHS is about 15 percent.
   c. Clinical presentation: Disease presentation usually occurs 10–14 days after pharyngitis or 2 –3 weeks after pyoderma. Usually patients experience sudden onset of edema, oliguria, azotemia, gross hematuria, and hypertension. At the onset of disease, symptoms may be nonspecific, such as pallor, malaise, low grade fever, anorexia, and headache. Gross hematuria, tea colored urine, is present in 30–70 percent of all patients, whereas microscopic hematuria is present in all patients. Edema in PSGN results from retention of salt and water and is not often recognized by parents. Most patients have mild morning periorbital edema. Hypertension is found in up to 70 percent of hospitalized patients due to salt and water retention. It is usually mild, but it can be severe. Hypertensive encephalopathy can be found in 0.5–10 percent of hospitalized patients. The children may manifest seizures, hemiparesis, or aphasia due to sudden elevations in blood pressure. Acute renal failure, hyperkalemia, congestive heart failure, and pulmonary edema are other serious complications in PSGN.
   d. Diagnosis: Proteinuria and hematuria are found in almost all patients with PSGN. The presence of an active urinary sediment with red blood cell casts and dysmorphic red blood cells are consistent with glomerular origin. A mild dilution anemia may be seen at the onset. Antistreptolysin O antigens should be present in cases of PSGN. The streptozyme test, which measures five different streptococcal antibodies, is positive in more than 95 percent of patients with PSGN

due to pharyngitis, and about 80 percent of those with skin infections. Poststreptococcal glomerulonephritis is associated with marked depression of C3 due to activation of the alternative pathways, often with normal C4.

e. Treatment: Fluid and salt restriction are generally sufficient in preventing edema and hypertension. Sodium should be restricted to less than 1 g/day. A potassium restriction should be instituted to prevent hyperkalemia. Moderate hypertension should be treated with loop diuretics and oral antihypertensive drugs, such as calcium channel blockers. ACE-inhibitors should be avoided. In a hypertensive emergency, Labetalol or hydralzaline may be given IV. Antibiotic therapy is indicated if there are still signs of streptococcal infection or patients with positive throat or skin cultures. Immunosupressive therapy is not indicated because the disease is self-limiting.

II. Rapidly Progressive Glomerulonephritis (RPGN)

1. A rapidly progressive glomerulonephritis is an uncommon presentation of many common nephrological disorders. Rapidly progressive glomerulonephritis is characterized by an active urinary sediment with progressive loss of renal function over days to months with glomerular crescents on renal biopsy. The more common causes are listed below.

   a. Membranoproliferative glomerulonephritis (MPGN):
      i. Pathogenesis: Membranoproliferative glomerulonephritis is characterized by mesangial proliferation and thickening of the peripheral glomerular basement membrane (GBM). It can occur as primary (idiopathic) or secondary forms. There are classically three types that are distinguished based on electron microscopy findings from renal biopsy.
      ii. Epidemiology: Primary MPGN is most common in older children and adolescents. Both male and female children are equally affected.
      iii. Clinical presentation: Type I MPGN usually has a slow, progressive course with remissions and exacerbations. It most commonly presents after 8 years of age initially with a nephritic pattern, but eventual nephrotic. Type II MPGN (dense deposit disease) present in young adulthood, with the vast majority of patients presenting less than 20 years of age. Secondary causes of MPGN are associated with a variety of diseases, but most commonly present with cryoglobulinemia, Hepatitis C, and Hepatitis B.

   b. Vasculitis/Primary glomerulonephritis
      i. A variety a vasculitidies and primary renal diseases are associated with RPGN in children including lupus nephritis, Henoch Schonlein Purpura (HSP), IgA nephrits, pauci-immune diseases including granulomatosis with polyangitis (formerly Wegener's

glomerulonephritis) and microscopic polyangitis, and Goodpastures syndrome or anti-GBM disease. These conditions are frequently associated with systemic manifestions such as rash, fever, pulmonary hemorrhage, joint complaints or malaise. A serologic evaluation is indicated including ANA, Anti-dna, ANCA, complements, quantitative immunoglobulins and anti-GBM antibody. A renal biopsy is needed to both confirm the diagnosis and assess the extent of disease. Emperic therapy with pulse methyprednisilone is indicated if RPGN is suspected pending the results of serologic testing and renal biopsy results.

c. Acute Tubulointerstitial Nephritis (ATIN)

   i. Pathogenesis: ATIN is characterized by interstitial cellular infiltrates, sparing the vessels and glomeruli. It is primarily a T-cell infiltration with some macrophages and plasma cells. An impressive number of eosinophils may be present. Antimicrobials and non-steroidal anti-inflammatory drugs (NSAIDs) are most commonly implicated.

   ii. Epidemiology: Acute injury to the renal interstium accounts for 5–15 percent of all cases of acute or chronic renal failure. In pediatric patients, ATIN accounts for 7 percent of acute renal failure in the pediatric setting, but in adults, the incidence is closer to 10 to 25 percent.

   iii. Clinical presentation: The classic presentation of drug-induced ATIN is fever, eosinophilia, and rash, but this is absent in more than 70 percent of patients. Patients complain of flank pain from interstitial edema causing renal enlargement.

   iv. Diagnosis: Often made clinically, but renal biopsy will confirm the diagnosis. Urine microscopy may reveal tubular epithelial cells and sterile pyuria. Urinary eosinophils are thought to be specific, but not sensitive for TIN. Nephromegaly can be seen on a renal sonogram.

   v. Treatment: Remove the suspected offending agent. Most cases are self-limited and clinically silent. Steroids may be indicated in severe/refractory cases, but a renal biopsy should confirm the diagnosis to direct therapy.

Congenital disorders of the kidney

I. Hydronephrosis

   a. Epidemiology: The widespread use of prenatal ultrasonography and improvements in technology have increased the detection of urinary structural changes, which are now discovered in 1 percent of pregnancies, of which more than 50 percent demonstrate hydronephrosis.

II. Posterior urethral valves (PUV)
   a. Epidemiology: Posterior uretheral valves are the most common cause of neonatal lower urinary tract obstruction in males. This abnormality occurs solely in males.
   b. Clinical presentation: Often posterior urethral valves are associated with other severe anomalies such as prune belly syndrome, cloacal anomalies, or VACTERL syndrome. Presentation is variable depending on the degree of obstruction. In severe cases, the patient may have an intra-abdominal mass, representing an enlarged kidney, and it would be difficult to pass a catheter. Patients can present with failure to thrive, urinatry tract infections, or acutely ill with AKI and severe electorolyte abnormalities such as hyponatremia, hyerkalemia, acidosis, hyperphosphatemia and hypocaclemia.
   c. Diagnosis: A renal sonogram typically demonstrates hydroureteronephrosis and may demonstrate a thickened and trabeculated bladder. The diagnosis is best made with a fluoroscopy voiding cystourethrogram and confirmed by cystoscopy.
   d. Treatment: Relief of the obstruction by cystoscopic ablation of the valves is critical in managing posterior urethral valves. Prognosis and intervention is variable, often depending on the degree of obstruction. Patients often have high output renal failure and require greater than standard maintenance fluids. A low solute infant formula, such as Similac PM 60/40, should be used once feeds are initiated. Careful monitoring for acidosis is necessary because the obstruction can cause tubular damage, resulting in renal tubular acidosis.

III. Prune belly syndrome
   a. Epidemiology: This is most commonly seen in males, but rarely seen in females.
   b. Clinical presentation: Prune belly syndrome is characterized by the underdevelopment of the abdominal wall muscles, hydroureters, hydronephrosis, and undescended testes. This syndrome presents with bilateral hydronephrosis and hydroureters with a large distended bladder and a wrinkled appearance to the abdominal wall. Postnatal renal failure is prominent and the patients also have pulmonary problems that lead to increased morbidity.
   c. Diagnosis: Clinical presentation.

IV. Ureteropelvic junction obstruction (UPJ)
   a. Clinical presentation: Patients are often asymptomatic and noted to have hydronephrosis on ultrasonography.
   b. Diagnosis: MAG3 furosemide renal scan.

V. Multicystic Dysplasic Kidney (MCDK)
   a. Clinical presentation: Patients with MCDK often are diagnosed on prenatal ultrasound or by palpable abdominal/flank mass shortly after

birth. Findings are most often unilateral. Up to 0.1 percent will have hypertension.
   b. Diagnosis: Renal ultrasonography.
   c. Treatment: Evaluation of the contralateral urinary tract is recommended because 25 percent of patients will have some abnormality on the contralateral side. Contralateral abnormalities include: hypoplasia, VUR, and UPJ obstruction. UPJ obstruction of the contralateral side can be seen in 5–10 percent of cases.

VI. Nephronophthisis (NPHP)
   a. Etiology: Familial disease characterized by autosomal recessive inheritance with a defect in urinary concentrating capacity. Gene defects in NPHP are responsible for the pathogenesis.
   b. Epidemiology: Terminal renal failure is reached between 7 and 29 years of age with median onset at 13.1 years of age.
   c. Clinical presentation: Children often present short stature and advance renal failure in early adolescents. The defect in urinary concentrating capacity results in symptoms of polyuria, resulting in enuresis and polydypsia. They often have no hypertension or proteinuria with a benign urinary sediment. Anemia is often out of proportion to degree of renal impairment.
   d. Diagnosis: Kidney biopsy or genetic testing is diagnostic.
   e. Treatment: Ultimately, patients with nephronophthisis will require kidney transplantation.

Nephrotic syndrome

I. Idiopathic nephrotic syndrome (INS)
   a. Pathogenesis: Evidence supports a role for T-cell activation and the secretion of an unknown permeability factor, but the exact method of pathogenesis remains unknown. Although no infectious agent has been identified as inducing nephrotic syndrome, there is an identifiable viral prodrome in about 50 percent of relapse cases.
   b. Epidemiology: The annual incidence of nephrotic syndrome is 2 to 7 per 100,000 children below the age of 16 with a prevalence of 16 per 100,000 children. The incidence is higher in Asian, African-American, and Arab children. The most common cause of nephrotic syndrome in children is minimal change disease, which is most often steroid responsive. Steroid resistant forms of nephritic syndromes are usually due to the focal segmental glomerulosclerosis (FSGS), mesangial hypercellularity, and membranous nephropathy. Steroid sensitive nephrotic syndrome is more common in boys than girls at a 2:1 ratio with peak incidence between 1 and 4 years, but the disparity disappears by adolescence. Steroid sensitive nephrotic syndrome is less common in

African and African- American children. In the past two decades, the proportion of children with steroid sensitive INS is falling.

c. Clinical presentation: 30–50 percent of cases are preceded by an upper respiratory tract infection. Most common symptoms include periorbital edema, ankle edema, but the spectrum can extend to include pleural effusions, scrotal/labial edema, and ascites. Some children have serious infections at presentation, particularly spontaneous bacterial peritonitis. Five to 20 percent of children present with hypertension.

d. Diagnosis: Edema, proteinuria > 40 mg/m^2/hr or protein/creatinine ratio > 2.0, and hypoalbuminemia (<2.5 mg/100mL). A urinalysis usually shows 3–4+ proteinuria. Microscopic hematuria may be present at diagnosis in 20–30 percent of children, but rarely persists and macroscopic hematuria occurs in less than 1 percent of steroid responsive INS. Renal function is generally normal, although serum creatinine may be elevated due to intravascular depletion at presentation. Elevated cholesterol and triglycerides are elevated while the child is nephrotic. Total calcium levels appear low due to hypoalbuminemia, but ionized calcium levels are normal. Kidney biopsy will help distinguish between causes of nephrotic syndrome, although podocyte fusion is universally appreciated. A renal biopsy is typically reserved for those children who have had a poor response to steroids, being either steroid resistant, steroid dependent, or frequently relapsing. A renal biopsy may be indicated prior to the initiation of steroids in an older adolescent, in whom the minimal change disease is a less likely diagnosis.

e. Treatment: Corticosteroids are the treatment of choice for INS. At presentation, children receive prednisone 2 mg/kg/d or 60 mg/m2/day (maximum 60 mg) divided twice daily for 4–6 weeks. If a remission has occurred, steroids are then reduced to 1.5 mg/kg or 40 mg/m^2 (maximum 40 mg) on alternate days for another 4–6 weeks, and then discontinued. In cases of severe edema (symptomatic ascites, pleural effusions, severe scrotal or labial edema), 25 percent albumin infusions followed by furosemide can be used to assist in diuresis. Albumin infusions should be used with caution as it can produce severe hypertension and result in pulmonary edema on occasion.

II. Congenital nephrotic syndrome (CNS)

a. Pathogenesis: Most commonly, a genetic cause, with the majority of mutation in the gene encoding nephrin, a podocyte slit diaphragm protein. This is most commonly an autosomal recessive disorder with variable penetrance.

i. Congenital nephrotic syndrome of Finnish type: Autosomal recessive inheritance with mutation in NPHS1 gene that encodes for nephrin.

ii. Recessive familial nephrotic syndrome: Autosomal recessive inheritance with mutation in NPHS2 gene that encodes for podocin.

    iii. Denys-Drash syndrome: Autosomal dominant inheritance with mutation in WT1 gene.

    iv. Frasier syndrome: Autosomal dominant inheritance with mutation in WT1 gene.

b. Clinical presentation: Nephrotic syndrome appearing in the first three months of life.

    i. Congenital nephrotic syndrome of the Finnish type: These children are usually born prematurely with a birth weight of 1500–3000 gm, with the placenta weighing over 25 percent of the birth weight. Proteinuria begins in utero and can be detected at birth. Congenital nephrotic syndrome should be suspected prenataly if elevated alpha-fetoprotein (AFP) levels are found in maternal serum and amniotic fluid in the absence of neural tube malformations.

    ii. Denys-Drash syndrome: Characterized by nephrotic syndrome in the first month of life, male pseudohermaphroditism, gonadal dysgenesis, and development of Wilm's tumor (>90 percent of patients). There is rapid deterioration to end stage renal disease.

    iii. Frasier syndrome: Characterized by progressive glomerulopathy and male pseudohermaphroditism with late onset of proteinuria in early childhood and development of end stage renal disease in second or third decade of life. Low risk for developing nephrotic syndrome, but gonadoblastomata is frequently observed.

c. Diagnosis: Genetic testing can now be used to distinguish forms of CNS, and a renal biopsy is no longer indicated.

d. Treatment: There is no definitive treatment for CNS and it does not respond to immunosuppressive therapy as other forms of nephrotic syndrome of childhood. Therapy in the newborn period is primarily supportive, consisting of 25 percent albumin infusions, a hypercaloric diet, and thyroxin supplementation, as thyroid-binding globulin is lost in the urine. Some experts have recommended aspirin and dipyridamole, but it has been of no proven benefit. Angiotensin-converting enzyme (ACE) inhibitors and indomethicin have been used in some patients to reduce proteinuria. Time to progression to end stage renal disease is variable. A common practice is to perform bilateral nephrectomies and begin peritoneal dialysis to avoid complications from nephrotic syndrome. This is followed by renal transplantation when a suitable size and weight is achieved.

Hypertension

Hypertensive children are more likely to have an identifiable cause of hypertension than adults. This is particular so in children who present with a hypertensive urgency or emergency. Similar to adults, hypertensive children are at risk for long-term target organ damage. Investigation of pediatric hypertension poses numerous problems including: measuring blood pressure and defining hypertension. Blood pressure measurements should ideally be performed after the patient is resting for five minutes, sitting upright, and with the arm at heart level. At least three measurements should be taken. The bladder cuff should cover 80–100 percent of the arm circumference and its width should be at least 38 percent of the arm circumference. Blood pressure measurements should be confirmed by ausculatory measurement. The initial evaluation of pediatric hypertension consists of renal function and biochemistries, a urinalysis and a renal ultrasound. Further testing may be indicated. The fourth report on diagnosis, evaluation, and treatment of high blood pressure in children and adolescents includes necessary charts for diagnosing hypertension based on age, gender, and height. Below are a discussion of the most common causes of primary hypertension in children that can result in a hypertensive urgency and emergency and its management,

I. Renal artery stenosis (RAS)
   a. Etiology: A compromised blood flow to one, both, or a portion of the kidneys.
   b. Clinical presentation: It is unusual to have mild hypertension in RAS. Patients can present asymptomatic or in hypertensive crisis. Some report history of headache, failure to thrive, or polyuria. Flank or abdominal bruits are not always present. It can be seen in children with neurofibromatosis or fibromuscular dysplasia or in infants with predisposing factors such as a history of umbilical vessel catheterization.
   c. Diagnosis: Although new techniques are available and used in adults, there is little experience in children. The gold standard continues to be formal intra-arterial angiography. The use of less invasive techniques such as CT and magnetic resonance angiography are desirable whenever the expertise is available and may have a greater role in the diagnosis. Renal sonogram with Doppler, enalaprilat renal scans, and peripheral plasma rennin and aldosterone level are relatively insensitive in detecting RAS.
   d. Treatment: ACE inhibitors are contraindicated if bilateral renal artery stenosis is present. Angioplasty of the vascular narrowing is desirable whenever possible, but this can be difficult in the small child.

II. Coarctation of the aorta
   a. Etiology: Narrowing of a segment of the aorta most commonly occurring in the juxtaductal area. Blood flow below the level of coarctation results in diminished renal blood flow and hypertension.
   b. Epidemiology: Accounts for nearly one-third of cases of hypertension in infancy.
   c. Clinical presentation: About 50 percent of cases are severe enough to cause symptoms in the neonatal period, but coarctation can go unrecognized for years. Delayed pulses compared to the lower extremities from upper extremities are often seen. Patients often have exercise intolerance, fatigue, and shortness of breath with exertion.

d. Diagnosis: Echocardiogram is the gold standard for diagnosing coarctation.
e. Treatment: Surgical correction is required.

III. Pheochromocytoma/paraganglioma
a. Etiology: A catecholamine-secreting tumor arising from chromaffin cells often originating in the adrenal medulla. Pheochromocytomas may be inherited as an autosomal dominant trait.
b. Epidemiology: 10 percent of pheochromocytomas occur in children, often between 6 and 14 years of age. They are more often on the right side, and, in more than 20 percent of affected children, the adrenal tumors are bilateral.
c. Clinical presentation: All patients have hypertension and unlike adults, children often have sustained hypertension. When there are paroxyms, patients usually complain of headache, palpitations, abdominal pain, and dizziness. Convulsion and other manifestations of hypertensive encephalopathy may occur.
d. Diagnosis: An elevated urinary catecholamine excretion or plasma free caecholamine is suggestive of a pheochromocytoma. Most tumors in the area of the adrenal glands can be visualized by ultrasonography, CT, or MRI. Radioactive Iodine Metaiodobenzylguanidine is taken up by chromaffin tissue and can be used to localize small tumors and the location of paragangliomas.
e. Treatment: Removal of tumor is curative. Preoperative consists of alpha blockade with phenoxybenzamine followed by beta blockade.

IV. Renal parenchymal disease
a. Etiology: The most common form of renal parenchymal injury associated with hypertension is pyelonephritic scarring/vesicoureteral reflux and various chronic and acute glomerulonephritides. In adolescents, hypertension may be the first manifestation of autosomal dominant polycystic kidney disease (PKD).
b. Epidemiology: Vesicoureteral reflux (VUR) nephropathy is responsible for 12–21 percent of all children with chronic renal failure and hypertension occurs in 10 to 30 percent of children with renal scarring.
c. Clinical presentation: Patients with renal scarring may present with no history of urinary tract infections or pyleonephritis and VUR nephropathy should not be ruled out by history alone. Patient commonly present with hypertension alone or with renal failure alone.
d. Diagnosis: Renal ultrasonography is an excellent first line evaluation and may reveal renal asymmetry in cases of scarring or cysts in PKD. Confirmation of renal scarring is established through nuclear medicine DMSA scan.
e. Treatment: The antihypertensive agents of choice for the treatment of renal parenchymal scarring are ACE inhibitors and angiotensin 2 receptor blockers.

V. Hypertensive urgencies and emergencies
   a. Definition: A hypertensive urgency is defined as severe elevation in blood pressure without evidence of severe symptoms of acute end organ damage. A hypertensive emergency is a severe elevation in blood pressure with life-threatening symptoms and or end organ injury.
   b. Management: Children with hypertensive urgencies can have their blood pressure initially managed with either intravenous bolus therapy or short active oral agent. Intravenous agents widely used in the management of hypertensive urgencies are Labetalol and hydralzine. Short acting oral agents that are effective are clonidine and isradipine. Children with hypertensive emergencies should managed with a continuous infusion of either Nicardipine, Nitroprusside or Labetalol in an ICU setting with an arterial line for continuous blood pressure monitoring.

Chapter 15

Acid-base disorders

John A Kellum

Overview

Increased intake, altered production or impaired/excessive excretion of acid or base leads to derangements in blood pH. With time, respiratory and renal adjustments correct the pH toward normality by altering the plasma levels of PCO_2 or strong ions (Na^+, Cl^-), and result in predictable changes in bicarbonate concentration that can also be used to characterize the disorder.

Increased intake

- Acidosis: chloride administration (e.g., saline), aspirin overdose.
- Alkalosis: $NaHCO_3$ administration, antacid abuse, buffered replacement fluid (hemofiltration).

Altered production

- Increased acid production: lactic acidosis, diabetic ketoacidosis.

Altered excretion

- Hypercapnic respiratory failure, permissive hypercapnia.
- Alkalosis: vomiting, large gastric aspirates, diuretics, hyperaldosteronism, corticosteroids.
- Acidosis: diarrhea, small bowel fistula, urethroenterostomy, renal tubular acidosis, renal failure, distal renal tubular acidosis, acetazolamide.

Approach to diagnosis

Alterations in acid-base balance produce characteristic patterns in arterial blood gases and plasma electrolytes. These changes can be used to make the diagnosis of respiratory, metabolic, or "complex" disorders (Table 15.1).

- Acidosis is associated with a decreased arterial plasma pH (<7.35), whereas alkalosis is associated with an increased arterial plasma pH (>7.45).
- Alterations not conforming to (within 2–3 units) the patterns described in Table 15.1 represent either laboratory error or complex (mixed) disorders.
- Laboratory error is best assessed by repeating the measurements.

Table 15.1 Simple acid-base disorders

Disorder	SBE (mEq/L)	pCO2 (mm Hg)	HCO3 (mmol/L)
Metabolic acidosis	≤ −5	40 + SBE	≤ 20
Metabolic alkalosis	≥ 5	40 + (0.6 × SBE)	≥ 28
Respiratory acidosis (chronic)	0 ± 4 0.4 × (pCO_2 −40)	>45	= [(pCO_2 −40)/10] + 24 = [(pCO_2 − 40)/3] + 24
Respiratory alkalosis (chronic)	0 ± 4 0.4 × (pCO_2 −40)	<35	= 24 − [(40 −pCO_2)/5] = 24 − [(40−pCO_2)/2]

Management

General management principles
- Correct (where possible) the underlying cause, for example, hypoperfusion.
- NaCl infusion for vomiting-induced alkalosis; insulin, Na^+ and K^+ in diabetic ketoacidosis.
- Correct pH in specific circumstances only, for example, $NaHCO_3$ in renal failure.
- Avoid large volume saline-based fluids. Consider lacted Ringer's solution or hetastarch in balanced electrolyte solution (Hextend) for fluid resuscitation.

Management with renal replacement therapy
- Acid-base abnormalities may be caused by improper use of renal replacement therapy (RRT) (e.g., during citrate anticoagulation) and are amenable to correction with RRT.
- Correction of plasma pH occurs because of change in plasma strong ion difference and to a small extent, change in weak acid concentration.
- Avoid "over correction" of acid-base abnormalities particularly in cases of metabolizable acid anions (e.g., lactate, ketones)—see metabolic acidosis.

A reduced arterial blood pH with a reduced strong ion difference and a base deficit >2 mEq/l. Outcome in critically ill patients has been linked to the severity and duration of metabolic acidosis and hyperlactatemia.

Metabolic acidosis

Causes
- Lactic acidosis. Can be due to tissue hypoperfusion, for example, circulatory shock. The anion gap (or strong ion gap) is increased with lactic and other

organic acids, and poisons. Anaerobic metabolism contributes in part to this metabolic acidosis; however, other cellular mechanisms are involved and may be more important. May be seen with increased muscle activity (e.g., postseizure, respiratory distress). Lung lactate release seen in acute lung injury. High, sustained levels suggest tissue necrosis, for example, bowel, muscle.

- Hyperchloremia, for example, excessive saline infusion.
- Ketoacidosis—high levels of β-hydroxybutyrate and acetoacetate related to uncontrolled diabetes mellitus, starvation, and alcoholism.
- Renal failure—accumulation of organic acids, for example, sulphuric.
- Drugs—in particular, aspirin (salicylic acid) overdose, acetazolamide (carbonic anhydrase inhibition), ammonium chloride. Vasopressor agents may be implicated, possibly by inducing regional ischemia or, in the case of epinephrine, accelerated glycolysis.
- Ingestion of poisons, for example, paraldehyde, ethylene glycol, methanol.
- Cation loss, for example, severe diarrhea, small bowel fistulae, large ileostomy losses.

Causes of lactic acidosis

- Sepsis.
- Acute lung injury.
- Diabetes mellitus.
- Drugs, for example, phenformin, metformin, and alcohols.
- Circulatory shock, for example, septic shock, hemorrhage, heart failure.
- Glucose-6-phosphatase deficiency.
- Hematological malignancy.
- Hepatic failure.
- Renal failure.
- Short bowel syndrome (D-lactate).
- Thiamine deficiency.

Clinical features

- Dyspnea.
- Hemodynamic instability.
- A rapidly increasing metabolic acidosis (over minutes to hours) is not due to renal failure. Other causes, particularly severe tissue hypoperfusion, sepsis, or tissue necrosis should be suspected when there is associated systemic deterioration.

General Management

- The underlying cause should be identified and treated where possible.
- Support ventilation (increase minute volume in controlled mechanical ventilation) to help normalize the arterial pH.

- Reversal of the metabolic acidosis is generally an indication of successful therapy. An increasing base deficit suggests that the therapeutic maneuvers in operation are either inadequate or wrong.
- The benefits of buffers such as Carbicarb and THAM (tris-hydroxymethyl-aminomethane) remain unproved.

RRT Management

- Urgent RRT may be necessary, particularly if renal function is also impaired.
- Lactate and ketones are easily removed by CRRT but they are also metabo-lized rapidly once the underlying metabolic derangement is reversed. CRRT is rarely the primary therapy for lactic or ketoacidosis.
- Hyperchloremia does not self-correct in a patient with anuric renal failure. Apart from diet, GI losses and intracellular shifts, the kidney is the primary regulator of plasma electrolytes.
- Continuous renal replacement therapy (CRRT) is effective in correcting hyperchloremic acidosis.

Metabolic alkalosis

An increased arterial blood pH with an increased strong ion difference and base excess >2mEq/l can be caused either by loss of anions or gain of cations. Because the kidney is usually efficient at regulating the strong ion difference, persistence of a metabolic alkalosis usually depends on either renal impairment or a diminished extracellular fluid volume with severe depletion of K^+ resulting in an inability to reabsorb Cl^- in excess of Na^+.

- The patient is usually asymptomatic though, if spontaneously breathing, will hypoventilate.
- A metabolic alkalosis will cause a left shift of the oxyhemoglobin curve, reducing oxygen availability to the tissues.
- If severe (pH > 7.6), may result in encephalopathy, seizures, altered coronary arterial blood flow, and decreased cardiac inotropy.

Causes

- Loss of total body fluid, Cl^-, usually due to:
- diuretics.
- large nasogastric aspirates, vomiting.
- Secondary hyperaldosteronism with KCl depletion.
- Use of hemofiltration replacement fluid containing excess buffer (e.g., lactate).
- Renal compensation for chronic hypercapnia. This can develop within 1–2 weeks. Although more apparent when the patient hyperventilates or is hyper-ventilated to normocapnia, an overcompensated metabolic alkalosis can oc-casionally be seen in the chronic state (i.e., a raised pH in an otherwise stable long- term hypercapnic patient).

- Excess administration of sodium bicarbonate.
- Excess administration of sodium citrate (large blood transfusion).
- Drugs, including laxative abuse, corticosteroids.
- Rarely, Cushing's, Conn's, Bartter's syndrome.

Management

- Replacement of fluid, Cl^- (i.e., give 0.9 percent saline) and K^+ losses are often sufficient to restore acid–base balance.
- With distal renal causes related to hyperaldosteronism, addition of spirono-lactone can be considered.
- Active treatment is rarely necessary. If so, administer 150 mL of 1.0 N HCl in 1 L sterile water using a central line. Infuse at a rate not greater than 1ml/kg/hr. Alternatives include ammonium chloride PO or if volume overloaded with intact renal function, acetazolamide 500 mg IV or PO q8h.
- Compensation for a long-standing respiratory acidosis, followed by correction of acidosis, for example, with mechanical ventilation, will lead to an uncompensated metabolic alkalosis. This usually corrects with time, though treatments such as acetazolamide can be considered. Mechanical "hypoventilation," that is, maintaining hypercapnia, can also be considered.

Respiratory acid-base disturbances are common in critically ill patients and represent abnormal increases or decreases in ventilation compared to patient needs.

Respiratory disorders

Classification

- Respiratory acidosis—excess CO_2 production and/or inadequate excretion.
- Respiratory alkalosis—reduction in pCO_2 due to increased ventilation relative to production.

Causes

Respiratory acidosis

- Central hypoventilation (e.g. decreased mental status, excess narcotic).
- Chronic obstructive lung disease ± acute exacerbation.
- Acute lung disease.
- Ventilation-perfusion (VQ) mismatch (e.g., pulmonary embolism).
- Increased CO_2 production with fixed ventilation (e.g., fever, shivering, seizures).

Respiratory alkalosis

- Hyperventilation with normal lungs (e.g., anxiety, salicylate intoxication).
- Hyperventilation due to hypoxemia (e.g., asthma exacerbation).
- Decreased CO_2 production with fixed ventilation (e.g., hypothermia, chemical paralysis on mechanical ventilation).

Management

- Treat underlying condition.
- Adjust ventilation to achieve appropriate pCO_2.

Respiratory acidosis

- Invasive or noninvasive mechanical ventilation.
- Increase minute ventilation (respiratory rate and/or tidal volume).
- Increase expiratory time when using advanced forms of ventilation.

Respiratory alkalosis

- Increase sedation, anti-anxiety therapy, or delirium management.
- Rarely: increase dead space in ventilator circuit.

Chapter 16

Electrolyte disorders

John A. Kellum

Electrolyte disorders are brought about either by electrolyte losses or by abnormalities in renal or gastrointestinal tract function leading to abnormal handling of electrolytes. Rarely electrolyte imbalance is brought about by exogenous administration, either enteral or parenteral. Electrolyte disorders can be life threatening.

Electrolyte losses

• Large nasogastric aspirate, vomiting	Na^+, Cl^-
• Sweating	Na^+, Cl^-
• Polyuria	Na^+, Cl^-, K^+, Mg^{2+}
• Diarrhea	Na^+, Cl^-, K^+, Mg^{2+}
• Ascitic drainage	Na^+, Cl^-, K^+

Dysnatremias

In general, dysnatremias that develop slowly should be treated slowly, whereas rapidly occurring dysnatremias demand rapid correction. Severe symptoms also require rapid treatment, although correction will be partial, at first, in the case of chronic conditions. Finally, volume status should be considered in the treatment plan.

Hypernatremia

Hypernatremia is manifest by thirst, lethargy, coma, seizures, muscular tremor, and rigidity, and an increased risk of intracranial hemorrhage. Thirst, usually occurs when the plasma sodium rises 3–4 mmol/L above normal. Lack of thirst is associated with central nervous system disease.

Rate of correction
- If hyperacute (<12 hour), correction should be rapid.
- Otherwise, aim for gradual correction of plasma sodium levels (over 1–3 days), particularly in chronic cases (>2 days' duration), to avoid cerebral edema

through sudden lowering of osmolality. A rate of plasma sodium lowering <0.7 mmol/h has been suggested.

Low or normal total-body Na (water loss)

- Reduce Na concentration in IV fluids (including replacement fluid and/or dialysate if receiving RRT).
- Water replacement PO may be given in addition to changes in IV fluids.
- Even fluid balance (or even fluid gain with replacement fluid) until total-body water is normalized.
- If central diabetes insipidus (CDI): restrict salt and give thiazide diuretics. Complete CDI will require desmopressin (10 µg bid intranasally or 1–2 µg bid IV), whereas partial CDI may require desmopressin but often responds to drugs that increase the rate of ADH secretion or end-organ responsiveness to ADH, for example, chlorpropamide, hydrochlorthiazide.
- If nephrogenic DI: manage by a low salt diet and thiazides. High-dose desmopressin may be effective. Consider removal of causative agents, for example, lithium.

Increased total-body Na (Na gain)

- Reduce Na concentration in IV fluids (including replacement fluid and/or dialysate if receiving RRT).
- Fluid removal targeted at achieving even or, if hypervolemia, net negative fluid balance.

Causes of hypernatremia

Type	Etiology	Urine
Low total body Na	Renal losses: diuretic excess, osmotic diuresis (glucose, urea, mannitol). Extra-renal losses: excess sweating.	$[Na^+]$ >20 mmol/L iso- or hypotonic $[Na^+]$ <10 mmol/L hypertonic
Normal total body Na	Renal losses: diabetes insipidus. Extra-renal losses: respiratory and renal insensible losses.	$[Na^+]$ variable hypo-, iso- or hypertonic $[Na^+]$ variable hypertonic
Increased total body Na	Conn's syndrome, Cushing's syndrome, excess NaCl, hypertonic $NaHCO_3$	$[Na^+]$ >20 mmoL/liso- or hypertonic

Hyponatremia

Hyponatremia may cause nausea, vomiting, headache, fatigue, weakness, muscular twitching, obtundation, psychosis, seizures, and coma. Symptoms depend on the rate as well as the magnitude of fall in the plasma $[Na^+]$.

Rate and degree of correction

• Rate and degree of correction depend on how rapidly the condition has developed and whether the patient is symptomatic. Hyponatremia that has developed over more than 48 hours is considered "chronic."

• In *chronic asymptomatic* hyponatremia, correction should not exceed 4 mmol/24 hours and the rate of correction should not exceed 0.3 mmol/L/hour.

• In *chronic symptomatic* (e.g., seizures, coma) hyponatremia, correction should be 1–1.5 mmol/L/hour until symptoms resolve; then correct as per asymptomatic cases.

• In *acute* hyponatraemia (< 48 hours), the ideal rate of correction is controversial, though elevations in plasma Na^+ can be faster, but <20 mmol/L/day.

• A plasma Na^+ of 120 mmol/L is a reasonable target for initial correction of symptomatic patients with chronic hyponatremia. Attempts to achieve eunatremia rapidly should be avoided.

• Neurological complications, for example, central pontine myelinolysis, are related to the degree of correction and (in chronic hyponatraemia) the rate. Premenopausal women are at highest risk for this complication.

Extracellular fluid (ECF) volume excess

• If symptomatic (e.g., seizures, agitation), 100 mL aliquots of hypertonic (1.8 percent) saline can be given, checking plasma levels every 2–3 hours.

• If symptomatic and edematous, fluid removal on CRRT can be provided in addition to hypertonic saline. Check plasma levels every 2–3 hours. With custom replacement fluid or dialysate, the Na concentration can be increased somewhat, but hypertonic dialysis or replacement fluid is not recommended.

• If not symptomatic, restrict water to 1–1.5 L/day. If hyponatremia persists, consider inappropriate ADH (SIADH) secretion.

Extracellular fluid volume (ECF) depletion

• If symptomatic (e.g., seizures, agitation), give isotonic (0.9 percent) saline. Consider hypertonic (1.8 percent) saline initially especially if acute.

• If asymptomatic, use isotonic (0.9 percent) saline.

• Maintain even fluid balance on CRRT.

Syndrome of Inappropriate ADH secretion (SIADH)

• SIADH is likely when the following are all present:
  • Hyponatremia.
  • Hypoosmolality.
  • Urine osmolality > 100 mosmol.
  • Urine Na > 40 meq/L are all present.

- Abnormal acid-base and potassium balance can confound the picture and mimic mild SIADH.
- Treatment
- If urine osmolality < 300 mosmol, isotonic saline is the first line of therapy.
  - Salt given in conjunction with a loop diuretic may be effective if the urine osmolality can be reduced.
  - For refractory cases, Conivaptan, 20 mg loading dose, followed by a continuous infusion of either 40 or 80 mg/day for 4 days has been shown to be effective. Monitor serum Na concentrations frequently and avoid rapid correction (see earlier).

General points

- Equations that calculate excess water are unreliable. It is safer to monitor plasma sodium levels closely.
- Hypertonic saline may be dangerous, especially in the elderly and those with impaired cardiac function.
- Use isotonic solutions for reconstituting drugs, parenteral nutrition, and so forth (i.e., avoid hypotonic fluids).
- Hyponatremia may intensify the cardiac effects of hyperkalemia.
- A true hyponatremia may occur with a normal osmolality in the presence of abnormal solutes, for example, ethanol, ethylene glycol, glucose.

Causes of hyponatremia

Type	Etiology	Urine [Na⁺]
ECF volume depletion	Renal losses: diuretic excess, osmotic diuresis (glucose, urea, mannitol), renal tubular acidosis, salt-losing nephritis, mineralocorticoid deficiency.	>20 mmol/L
	Extrarenal losses: vomiting, diarrhoea, burns, pancreatitis	<10 mmol/L
Modest ECF volume excess (no edema)	Water intoxication (NB postoperative, TURP syndrome), inappropriate ADH secretion, hypothyroidism, drugs (e.g., carbamazepine, chlorpropamide), glucocorticoid deficiency, pain, stress.	>20 mmol/L
	Acute and chronic renal failure.	>20 mmol/L
ECF volume excess (edema)	Nephrotic syndrome, cirrhosis, heart failure.	<10 mmol/L

Causes of inappropriate ADH secretion

- Neoplasm, for example, lung, pancreas, lymphoma.
- Most pulmonary lesions.
- Most central nervous system lesions.
- Surgical and emotional stress.

- Glucocorticoid and thyroid deficiency.
- Idiopathic.
- Drugs, for example, chlorpropamide, carbamazepine, narcotics.

Potassium

Both K^+ and Mg^{2+} are primarily intracellular cations; their total-body concentrations depend on the balance between intake and excretion, whereas their plasma concentrations are determined by total body stores as well as by their distribution across cell membranes. In the case of K^+, plasma pH and $[Na^+]$ also affect the plasma concentration. Excretion is primarily controlled by the kidneys although both cations are excreted in the feces as well.

Hyperkalemia

Hyperkalemia may cause dangerous arrhythmias including cardiac arrest. Arrhythmias are more closely related to the rate of rise of potassium than the absolute level. Clinical features such as paraesthesia and areflexic weakness are not clearly related to the degree of hyperkalemia but usually occur after ECG changes (tall "T" waves, flat "P" waves, prolonged PR interval and wide QRS).

Causes

- Reduced renal excretion (e.g., renal failure, adrenal insufficiency, diabetes, potassium sparing diuretics).
- Intracellular potassium release (e.g., acidosis, rapid transfusion of old blood, cell lysis including rhabdomyolysis, hemolysis, and tumor lysis).
- Potassium poisoning.

Management

Continuous renal replacement therapy is effective in removing K+ although standard hemodialysis can remove K+ faster. Ancillary therapy may also be required, particularly in emergency situations (see chapter 9).

Hypokalemia

Typical manifestations of hypokalemia include:

- Arrhythmias (SVT, VT, and Torsades de Pointes).
- ECG changes (ST depression, "T" wave flattening, "U" waves).
- Constipation.
- Ileus.
- Weakness.

Causes

- Inadequate intake.
- Gastrointestinal losses (e.g., vomiting, diarrhea, fistula losses).

- Renal losses (e.g., diabetic ketoacidosis, Conn's syndrome, secondary hyperaldosteronism, Cushing's syndrome, renal tubular acidosis, metabolic alkalosis, hypomagnesemia, drugs including diuretics, steroids, theophyllines).
- Hemofiltration losses.
- Potassium transfer into cells (e.g., acute alkalosis, glucose infusion, insulin treatment, familial periodic paralysis).

Management

Potassium replacement should be intravenous with ECG monitoring when there is a clinically significant arrhythmia (20 mmol over 30 minutes, repeated according to levels). Slower intravenous replacement (20 mmol over 1 hour) should be used where there are clinical features without arrhythmias. Oral supplementation (to a total intake of 80–120 mmol/day, including nutritional input) can be given when there are no clinical features.

Chapter 17

Management of the renal transplant patient in the ICU

Nirav Shah and Jerry McCauley

Among the great marvels of modern medicine are the advances of kidney transplantation for the treatment of end stage kidney disease (ESKD). The increasing numbers of patients with kidney transplantation bears witness to the successes in the field. Most recent estimates from UNOS-United Network for Organ Sharing estimates a prevalence of 150,000 kidney transplants with an estimated 16,000 done annually. Patients with kidney transplants are admitted to the ICU for reasons similar to those from the general population but at a higher frequency due to the nature of immunosuppressants and their effects: infections, malignancies, and cardiovascular disease. The focus of the chapter will be the management of the fresh transplant recipient in the ICU setting.

The majority of kidney transplant recipients can be monitored in non-ICU medical floor settings skilled in the postoperative management of highly variable blood pressures, fluid and electrolyte management in an immunosuppressed individual. However, there are many special situations in which monitoring and management of these patients is better served in the ICU setting including: high risk cardiovascular disease, advanced pulmonary hypertension, brittle diabetics requiring insulin drips, tenuous volume overload and the setting of delayed or slow graft function (DGF/SGF), refractory hyper/hypotension, and with patients who are difficult to extubate from the OR and/or those in prolonged respiratory failure.

Management of transplant patients is, in many ways, similar to management of patients without kidney transplantation; however, increased awareness is required with particular aspects of their medical care due to the underlying medical co-morbidities associated with ESKD or to conditions associated with the transplantation process and use of transplant medications.

Delayed or slow graft function

Delayed or slow graft function (DGF/SGF) is defined as the need for dialysis within the first week posttransplantation or lack of decrease in serum creatinine after kidney transplantation. Etiology can be broken down into characteristics of donor organ and transplant process verses immune and nonimmune factors. Early detection can facilitate reversal in many cases (Table 17.1).

143

Table 17.1 Etiology of DGF/SGF

Factors	Diagnosis	Management
Donor related • Prolonged cold ischemia time (>24 hours) • Expanded criteria donor (HTN, elderly donor, elevated creatinine (Cr) at harvesting) • Donation after cardiac death, non-heart-beating donor • Donor death with ATN • Pediatric donor • Donor/recipient mismatch in size and gender	By history	Supportive treatment; Can give furosemide 80 mg IV for symptomatic overload, IVF challenge if not clinically overloaded; use RRT (HD/CRRT/PD) as clinically indicated
Surgical factors • Renal allograft vessel thrombosis/stenosis	Renal ultrasound with Doppler, nuclear perfusion scan	Surgical exploration and revision; thrombectomy percutaneous angioplasty of vessels
• Ureteral stenosis/leak	Renal ultrasound, pyelogram; *Ureteral stenosis:* no reduction in hydronephrosis despite foley placement. *Urinary leak:* Sending fluid sample for Cr value.. greater than serum Cr suggests urine leak)	Surgical exploration and revision; percutaneous nephrostomy; ureteral stent
Recipient factors Hypotension (hypovolemia, anemia, sepsis, cardiovascular)	Clinical diagnosis	Correction of underlying etiology
Immune mediated factors Acute vs. hyper-acute rejection	Clinical presentation, renal biopsy, transplant cross match, donor specific antibodies	*Hyper acute rejection* from preformed antibodies necessitates removal of allograft. *Acute cellular (ACR) vs antibody mediated rejection (AMR)* involves high dose steroids, thymoglobulin vs. IVIG, plasmapheresis depending on type/severity of rejection.
Recurrence of primary disease/i.e., focal segmental sclerosis (FSGS), thrombotic microangiopathy (TMA)	Clinical scenario, renal biopsy	Steroids, plasmapheresis and adjustment of immunosuppressants if TMA related to calcineurin inhibitors.

Cardiovascular disease

Besides infection and sepsis, cardiovascular disease is the leading cause of morbidity and mortality of transplant recipients in the perioperative and long-term setting. Incidence of clinically significant cardiovascular disease in ESKD patients approaches >50 percent, depending on the criteria used. Patient with ESKD have multiple traditional and nontraditional risk factors for cardiovascular disease including hypertension, proteinuria, anemia, left ventricular hypertrophy, hypercholesterolemia, dystrophic calcification, and uremic cardiomyopathy. Many therapeutic clinical studies on management of cardiovascular disease exclude patients with renal failure; therefore, evidence-based data are limited. However, management strategies used in non-renal-failure patients are used in this population. Preoperative cardiovascular stress tests and cardiac catheterization done routinely have a limited role in the perioperative cardiovascular management, and they are often trumped by patients' functional capacity and practices of high cardiovascular risk management (Table 17.2).

Pulmonary hypertension

Pulmonary hypertension (PH) is recognized in the general population at rates of 15/million, but it is seen at an astonishingly high rate of one-third of the ESKD population, depending on the modality and criteria used. A large contributor toward this phenomenon is that the ESKD population with HD is chronically volume overloaded. Other significant risk factors include: high output AV fistulas and shunting of blood, high incidence of left heart disease and valvular disease in the ESKD patient, dialysis alterations of mediators of vasoconstriction and vasodilatation and micro emboli with dialysis, and the high incidence of collagen vascular disease in this population. These patients have an increased odds ratio for allograft failure (4.0), and patient death (10) most commonly occurring from right ventricule failure, respiratory failure, and difficulty weaning.

Management strategies: Risk stratifying patients based on pre- and post-transplant Echo/right heart catheritization according to right ventricular and

Table 17.2 Steps to minimize cardiovascular complications
1. Use of perioperative and postoperative beta-blockers in high risk recipients
2. Avoid holding plavix if recent cardiovascular stent placement within 6 weeks for bare metal stent and within 1 year for drug eluting stent
3. Holding erythropoetin stimulating agent in perioperative setting to reduce risk of thrombosis because medication is also unlikely to be effective with acute inflammatory state and has increased risks for thrombosis, MI, death
4. Control of hypertension and HR with short-term SBP goals of 140 mmHg posttransplantation
5. No routine holding of statins, aspirin, or BP meds that are at high risk for withdrawal (clonidine, beta blockers) unless contraindications

pulmonary artery systolic pressures. Begin aggressive management of volume status, with diuretics and RRT as necessary. Finally one should consider early weaning trials, aggressive pulmonary toilets to minimize incidences of pneumonia, and adequate deep vein thrombosis (DVT) prophylaxis to prevent pulmonary emboli that can be disastrous in this population of patients.

Volume/electrolyte abnormalities

The pattern of electrolyte abnormalities seen in renal transplant recipients is highly dependent on allograft function and urine output. There is significant diuresis post-kidney transplantation, when urine outputs can reach 500–1000 cc/hour, especially after a living kidney donation, which can lead to hypovolemia. This massive volume loss can also result in severe electrolyte and acid-base derangements.

Volume management: Because large portions of the ESKD population have underlying pulmonary hypertension, left ventricular hypertrophy (LVH), valvular disease, coronary artery diease (CAD), underlying pulmonary disease, and sleep apnea, they are highly sensitive to fluid status and shifts. Depending on the clinical status postoperatively, intravenous fluids are usually matched based on urine outpatient and highly dependent on quality of allograft function. In general, during the first 24 hours, the first 300 cc/hour of urine output is matched at a rate of 1:1 of isotonic IVF per urine output. Outputs greater than 300 cc/hour are matched at a rate of four-fifths of urine output, requiring careful nursing attention of inputs and outputs.

Electrolytes disorders are highly dependent on allograft function and the medications used in transplantation (Table 17.3).

Table 17.3 Electrolytes disorders posttransplant

Electrolyte disorder	Goal	Treatment
Hyperkalemia: • Decreased excretion usually seen in patients with DGF/SGF • Increased intake (additive, transfusions) • Medication related, i.e., Type IV RTA • Transcellular shift (tissue destruction postsurgery, hemolysis, hyperglycemia, metabolic acidosis)	K =4–5 mMol/l	1. Check EKG to see if risk for cardiac arrhythmia, if EKG changes use IV calcium gluconate or calcium chloride for membrane stabilization 2. Withdraw/reduce offending medications if possible, i.e., ACE inhibitor, angiotensin receptor blocker, bactrim 3. Increase intracellular shift (insulin +/-D50, beta agonist (albuterol), sodium bicarbonate (each IV amps = 50 meq HCO^3, or oral sodium bicarb onate tablets each 650 mg tab = 7 meq HCO^3 4. Removal of K from body: furosemide 80 mg IV and NS IVF to increase urine flow, mineralocorticoids such as florinef 0.1 mg po bid may help with RTA. **Avoid use of Kayexalate in patient with postop ileus due to risk of bowel perforation**

Table 17.3 (Continued)

Electrolyte disorder	Goal	Treatment
Hypokalemia: Commonly seen in patients with excessive postoperative diuresis and those with large GI losses		Repletion and recheck as often as necessary, IV or PO based on severity and NPO status. Important to correct underlying hypomagnesemia if present
Hypocalcemia: Common in patient with ESKD and reduced ability to activate vitamin D as well as those with history of surgical parathyroidectomy or equivalent medication cinacalcet/Sensipar, or large volume blood transfusion	Corrected Ca: 8–10 mg/dl	Confirm with ionized calcium and replace IV vs. PO calcium based on severity and presence of symptoms D/C on offending medications (e.g., cinacalcet, bisphosphonates). May require addition of activated vitamin D (i.e., calcitriol). May require repletion of concomitant hypomagnesemia with affects PTH release.
Hypercalcemia: Seen in patients with underlying hyperparathyroidism with ESRD		• DC of vitamin D and calcium-based phosphorous binders. Role of cinacalcet/sensipar. • May correct with a well functioning transplant. • Use of other agents include IVF/hydration+furosemide, calcitonin, and bisphophonates depends on severity and symptoms and underlying renal function.
Hyperphosphatemia: Seen in patients with DGF/SGF	3.5–5.0 mg/dl	Dietary modifications and use of phosphorous binders with meals. Examples calcium acetate (Phoslo), sevelamer (renagel), lanthanum (Fosrenol). If elevated Caxphos product discontinue vitamin D.
Hypophosphatemia: Seen commonly posttransplant as renal function now responding to endogenous PTH and those patients on CRRT for DGF		Can replete with oral or IV phos based on severity. In general, if <1.5 mg/dl, consider IV replacement. • When severe can contribute to muscular weakness, resp failure, rhabdomyolysis.
Hypomagnesemia Common post-kidney transplantation and include GI and urine magnesium losses aggravated by calcineurin inhibitors and large diuresis	1.6–2.0 mg/dl	Hypomagnesemia. Oral replacements include Mag Oxide, magnesium chloride, and magnesium gluconate. Dose often limited by diarrhea. Risk of hypomagnesemia includes hypocalcemia and cardiac arrhythmias. IV magnesium needed for severe hypomagnesemia <1.0 mg/dl.

Postoperative bleeding/hyper-coagulable state

Patients with ESKD have many risk factors for bleeding post-kidney transplantation, including uremia-induced platelet dysfunction; thrombocytopenia from bone marrow suppression from medications; and high prevalence of aspirin, plavix, and warfarin. Many patients with ESKD are on chronic anticoagulation for hypercoagulable states, and atrial fibrillation is seen in greater frequency in patients with collagen vascular disease and autoimmune conditions such as lupus and heart disease. These patients are urgently reversed with short-acting fresh frozen plasma (FFP) at the time of surgery; however, because the FFP has a shorter half-life than warfarin, they develop significant bleeding risks postoperatively and need to be monitored and corrected.

Conversely, many ESKD patients are hypercoagulable and have high risk of allograft vessel thrombosis in the postoperative period. They will need to have some form of anticoagulation started at soon as safely possible from the surgical hemostasis standpoint. With variable renal function posttransplant, unfractionated heparin may be preferable to low molecular weight heparin (LMWH) because its renal mode of elimination would make titration difficult in the postoperative setting with variable glomerular filtration rate (GFR).

Postoperative infections

It is not unusual for the recipient to have leucopenia in the posttransplant setting due to bone marrow and immune suppressing medications. The use of a lymphocyte depleting protocol with induction with alemtuzimab or thymoglobulin will exacerbate this process and require a battery of prophylaxis medication to reduce risks of developing infections in the short-term setting. The use of bone marrow stimulating agents to treat pancytopenia is controversial and requires balancing the risk/benefit of therapy. The majority of immediate posttransplant infections are bacterial related to wound, lung, urinary, and line infections. Donor cadaver culture may turn positive after kidney harvesting for which the recipients may require treatment and follow-up.

Viral infections are common in the immunocompromised leucopenic recipients, and are more common in cases in which there is donor/recipient mismatching or there is a history of viral infection and exposure. For example, patients who are cytomegalovirus (CMV) negative and who receive a CMV positive donor are at higher risk of developing CMV disease, and prophylaxis is warranted. Similar prophylaxis has been directed at patients with Epstein Barr virus. Prophylaxis has an important role in reducing the rate of primary infection and post-transplant malignancy (PTLD) in the future (Table 17.4).

Table 17.4 Routine prophylaxis posttransplantation

Agent	Properties	Dose and Duration	Notes
Bactrim SS Alternatives Dapsone, Pentamidine, atovaquone	UTI, PCP, nocardia, listeria, toxoplasmosis	QD to Q MWF, duration of 3 month– indefinitely, depending on risk factors	Adjust for GFR, can cause bone marrow suppression, hyperkalemia, elevated creatinine
Nystatin swish and swallow Alternatives Diflucan, voriconazole	Antifungal	5 cc QID for 3 months	Depends on risks/ presence of infection/level of immunosuppression. Interactions with calcineurin inhibitor.
Valgancyclovir Alternative acyclovir	Antiviral for CMV, EBV, HHV	3 months–1 year Depend on donor recipient mismatch	Need adjustment for renal function
Isoniazid plus B6	Anti Mycobacterium	6–9 months	Prophylaxis given in PPD positive recipients or donors. Need monitoring of LFT's.

Hypertension management

Although long-term management of blood pressure in renal transplant recipients with chronic kidney disease (CKD) goals may be <140/90, the short-term postoperative goals are not as rigid. Hypotension has risks of allograft vessel thrombosis in addition to usual risks. Care should be taken to monitor orthostatic blood pressure changes in these patients with hypovolemia and the inability of fresh kidneys to regulate volume status. Additionally, there is a high frequency of underlying neuropathy in patients with long-standing diabetes and kidney disease.

Patients tend to require less antihypertensive care with improved renal function and sodium and fluid handling posttransplantation. General principles include those shown in Table 17.5.

Transplant medications

The immunosuppression regimen is highly variable, and it centers specifically, with no generalized standard of care. Some centers use steroid sparing and use of induction regimens. Ideally the regimen is tailored to the individual patient, weighing the risk for rejection and toxicities from the medication, history of malignancy, and degree of HLA matching. It his helpful to know the side-effect profile, drug- dose targets, and mechanisms of action and drug interactions of the most commonly use medications in transplantation. See Tables 17.6 and 17.7.

Table 17.5 Principle of hypertension management in renal transplant recipient

Avoid tight control in patient with orthostatic hypotension from hypovolemia and neuropathy.

Holding ACE-I, and ARB until creatinine has stabilized may reduce frequency and need for HD for DGF and hyperkalemia.

Preference for dihydropyridine class of calcium channel blocker to counteract vasoconstriction caused by calcineurin inhibitors. Nondihydropyridine class of calcium channel blocker will raise calcineurin inhibitors levels.

Monitor for withdrawal of antihypertensive in postoperative setting such as beta-blocker or alpha blocker withdrawal.

Use of low-dose diuretics in patient with concomitant hyperkalemia as well as patients with volume overload.

Work up for secondary cause of hypertension such as renal allograft artery stenosis in patients with resistant hypertension and volume overload.

Table 17.6 Common drug interactions

Drug-drug Interactions

- Common drugs that *increase* calcineurin levels:
  - Allopurinol
  - Macrolides—Erythromycin, Clarithromycin
  - Ciprofloxacin
  - Azoles—Flucanazole
  - Nondihydropyridine calcium channel blockers (Verapamil, Diltiazem)
  - Protease inhibitors
  - Propofol
  - INH
  - Viagra
  - Select psychotropics, benzodiazepines
  - Lovastatin, simvastatin
  - Oral contraceptive
  - Grapefruit juice
  - Imipenem may increase CNS toxicity

- Common drugs that *decrease* calcineurin levels
  - Nafcillin
  - Rifampin
  - Seizure meds
  - Ticlid
  - St. John's wort, cat's claw, echinacea

Table 17.7 Common transplant medications

Drug	Dosing/Levels	Side Effects	Mechanism
Calcineurin inhibitors (CNIs)		Hyperkalemia, hyperuricemia, hypomagnesemia, Na retention, HUS	Prevents T cell proliferation. Blocks dephosphorylation of the nuclear factor of activated T cells which prevents transcription of cytokines (such as IL-2) and production of T cells.
Tacrolimus/FK506 (Prograf)	0.1mg/kg/d divided BID 12h trough 8–10ng/mL x 3mos, then 6–8	Alopecia, islet cell toxicity, neurotoxicity, HOCM, knee pain (try Nifedipine)	Inhibits phosphatase activity of calcineurin by binding with an immunophilin (FK binding protein).
Cyclosporine (CyA) (Sandimmune, Neoral, Gengraf, Eon, Sidmak)	IV is 1/3 PO dose. Formulations are NOT interchangeable. MC ~3–4mg/k/d, may need 10–20% less with microemulsion. 12-hour trough 200–300ng/mL x 3 mos, then 100–200. 2-hour peak (C2) levels may be better; 1000–1500 ng/mL x 6 mos, then 800–900 (if using TG/Campath induction, consider 800–1000 x 3 mos, then 400–600).	HTN, Hyperlipidemia, Hirsutism, Acne, gingival hyperplasia (can try flagyl 750 tid x 14d or azithro 500 mg qd x 3d for mild disease). Reversible leukoencephalopathy.	Forms a complex with an immunophilin (cyclophilin), which inhibits phosphorylation of calcineurin
Sirolimus (Rapamycin, Rapamune)	Loading dose 6–15 mg/d in 2 divided doses Levels should be 5–15 ng/ml. Half-life is 57 to 63 H; monitor after 5–7 days of stable therapy.	Cytopenias, ↑ lipids, HTN, edema, poor wound healing (not recommended for lung tx), hepatic artery thrombosis (not approved for liver tx), interstitial lung disease (may be useful in setting of KS), diarrhea, nausea	Arrests T cell cycle in G1-S phase, by inhibiting T cell proliferation induced by lymphokines. Binds to the FK binding protein complex then modulates activity of the rapamycin target protein

(continued)

Table 17.7 (Continued)

Drug	Dosing/Levels	Side Effects	Mechanism
Antimetabolites			
Azathioprine	2.5 mg/kg/d monitor thioguanine levels	Do NOT use with allopurinol (sig risk of Stevens-Johnson)	Imidazole derivative of 6-mercaptopurine; antagonizes purine metabolism and may inhibit synthesis of DNA, RNA, and proteins
Mycophenolate mofetil (MMF) (Cellcept) Mycophenolic acid (Myfortic)	MMF 500 mg–1g BID levels not currently monitored. Cellcept and Myfortic are NOT equivalent.	GI distress, HTN, ↑ lipids, pulmonary fibrosis (contraindicated with Lesch-Nyhan or Kelley Seegmiller)	Inhibitor of inosine monophosphate dehydrogenase (IMPDH), interfering with the de novo pathway of purine synthesis and DNA replication, producing cytostatic effects on T and B cells
Cyclophosphamide (Cytoxan)	Not known	Cytopenias, alopecia, GI distress, hemorrhagic cystitis, ovarian failure	Alkylating agent, prevents cell division by cross-linking DNA strands and decreasing DNA synthesis
Leflunomide (Arava)	(For treating CMV or BK virus) Loading dose: 100 mg daily for 5 days Usual dosage: after 5 days give 40–60 mg daily levels > or = 50 ug/ml < 80 ug/ml		Inhibits de novo pyrimidine (rUMP) synthesis at the level of the enzyme dihydro-orotate-dehydrogenase (DHODH)

Steroids		
Solumedrol Prednisone	5–7.5 mg/d for triple therapy	Metabolic, infections, osteoporosis, DM, HTN, poor wound healing	Inhibit production of T cell lymphokines, interferon, TNF and cause lymphocytes and macrophages to migrate from the circulation to lymph nodes

Antibody Preparations		
IVIG	500 mg/k/d x 4–7 d		decrease new antibody formation
Alemtuzumab (Campath)	30 mg IV over 2 hours once for induction		Binds to CD52 causing lysis of T cells, B cells, NK cells, macrophages
Antithymocyte Globulins • Thymoglobulin (derived from rabbit)	Premedicate with steroids, acetaminophen, and diphenhydramine *Induction:* 5mg/kg IV over 6 hours x 1 *Rejection:* 1.5 mg/kg x 7–14 days	Fevers, chills Myalgias, arthralgias, ↑WBC, ↑plts	Depletes lymphocytes via complement lysis or phagocytosis. Polyclonal IgG binds to multiple T cell epitopes
• Atgam (derived from horses)	*Rejection:* 15 mg/k/d x 7–14 days		

(continued)

Table 17.7 (Continued)

Drug	Dosing/Levels	Side Effects	Mechanism
Muromonab-CD3 (OKT3)	Premedicate with steroids, acetaminophen, and diphenhydramine 5 mg IV push for 10–14 days	Pulmonary edema. May result in titers of antimurine antibodies. If > 1:1000 may limit efficacy ↑HR, ↑↓ BP, ↑T, SOB, edema, chills, headache, rash, diarrhea, vomiting	Murine monoclonal antibody that binds CD3, prohibiting antigen recognition
Basiliximab (Simulect)	20 mg within 2 hours prior to transplant surgery, followed by a second 20 mg dose 4 days after transplantation	HTN, edema, ↑T, SOB, headache, acne, wound complications, ↑ lipids, hyperglycemia, ↑/↓ K, ↑ Phos	Inhibits T cell proliferation by blocking the IL-2 receptor
Daclizumab (Zenapax)	1 mg/kg infused over 15 minutes within 24 hours before transplantation	Chest pain, edema, ↑ HR, dizziness, ↑T, fatigue, headache, insomnia, thrombosis, abdominal pain, N/V, dysuria, oligura, ATN, pulmonary edema, lymphocele	Inhibits T cell proliferation by blocking the IL-2 receptor
Rituximab (Rituxan)	375 mg/m² per week × 4		Effect on CD20 pre-B and mature B-cells
Bortezomib (Velcade)	1.3 mg/m² or 1.5mg/kg × 4	Thrombocytopenia, GI	Effect is on proteosomes with action on mature plasma cells

Suggested readings

Bostom AD. Prevention of post-transplant cardiovascular disease—report and recommendations of an ad hoc group. *Am J Transplant.* 2002 Jul;2(6):491–500. PubMed PMID: 12118892.

Fishman JA. Infection in renal transplant recipients. *Semin Nephrol.* 2007 Jul;27(4):445–461. Review. PubMed PMID: 17616276.

Friedman GS. Hypercoagulable states in renal transplant candidates: impact of anticoagulation upon incidence of renal allograft thrombosis. *Transplantation.* 2001 Sep 27;72(6):1073–1078. PubMed PMID: 11579303.

Issa N. Pulmonary hypertension is associated with reduced patient survival after kidney transplantation. *Transplantation.* 2008 Nov 27;86(10):1384–1388. PubMed PMID: 19034007.

Pfeffer MA; TREAT Investigators. A trial of darbepoetin alfa in type 2 diabetes and chronic kidney disease. *N Engl J Med.* 2009 Nov 19;361(21):2019–2032. PubMed PMID: 19880844.

Ramakrishna G, Sprung J, Ravi BS, et al. Impact of pulmonary hypertension on the outcomes of noncardiac surgery: predictors of perioperative morbidity and mortality. *J Am Coll Cardiol.* 2005 May 17;45(10):1691–1699. PubMed PMID: 15893189.

Shaheen MF, Impact of recipient and donor nonimmunologic factors on the outcome of deceased donor kidney transplantation. *Transplant Proc.* 2010 Jan–Feb;42(1):273–276. PubMed PMID: 20172328.

Wang JH, Kasiske BL. Screening and management of pretransplant cardiovascular disease. *Curr Opin Nephrol Hypertens.* 2010 Nov;19(6):586–591. PubMed PMID: 20948378.

Endocrine and Metabolic Disease

Chapter 18

Diabetes mellitus

Eric A. J. Hoste

Diabetes mellitus (DM) is a metabolic disorder characterized by chronic hyper-glycemia, caused by defects of insulin secretion, insulin action, or a combination of these.

In 2007, 23.6 million patients or 7.8 percent of the population in the United States had DM. The prevalence of DM is increasing in recent years. Over the period 1980 to 2008 there was a 10.1 percent annual increase of the prevalence in the United States (http://www.cdc.gov/diabetes/statistics/prev/national/figper-sons.htm, accessed November 8th 2010). The prevalence of DM is higher in older patients. In patients over 60 years, who constitute approximately half of the ICU admissions, 23.1 percent of patients have DM. Other patient groups at risk for DM are patients with lower income, lower education, Hispanics, and African Americans. Patients with DM have a high risk for chronic complications such as cardiovascular disease, stroke, high blood pressure, blindness, kidney disease, and disorders of the nervous system. DM patients can also be admitted with acute diseae, such as acute hyperglycemic crisis and life-threatening acute complications such as diabetic keto-acidosis (DKA) and hyperglycemic hyperosmolar coma (HHC).

In addition, 25.9 percent of U.S. adults >20 years of age, and 35.4 percent of people >60 years of age, have impaired fasting glucose or prediabetes. These patients are at risk for increased blood glucose, a frequent complication in ICU patients, which may impact outcome.

Impact of DM and increased blood sugar on critical illness

Diabetes and critical illness

Diabetics who are admitted in the ICU are at greater risk for having more co-morbid conditions. This will result in more severe organ dysfunction, such as acute kidney injury (AKI) and need for renal replacement therapy (RRT), and hemodynamic instability. There are conflicting data about whether diabetes is associated with increased risk for infection and sepsis in ICU patients.

Despite greater co-morbidity, diabetes does not incur higher mortality in ICU patients when corrected for severity of illness.

Hyperglycemia and critical illness
Hyperglycemia at time of admission
Hyperglycemia at time of admission is, in most studies, associated with worse outcomes, especially in patients who are admitted with cardiovascular diagnoses such as myocardial infarction or stroke, but also in ICU patients. In general ICU patients, the association of admission hyperglycemia and increased mortality is present only in patients without a history of DM. However, in patients with acute coronary syndromes, this association is also present in diabetics in some studies.

This illustrates that hyperglycemia has different biological effects in diabetics and nondiabetics, and that these are even different in specific cohorts.

Strict glucose control or intensive insulin therapy
The concept of intensive insulin therapy was already developed 10-years ago by Van den Berghe and co-workers in Leuven, and has raised much discussion since. In their first single-center study in surgical ICU patients, intensive insulin therapy to maintian blood glucose < 110 mg/dL resulted in reduced morbidity and mortality. Further analysis of the results demonstrated that strict blood glucose control, rather than administration of insulin was the reason for the favorable effects. Since this first study, more than 30 additional studies were published on this concept. Most of these studies included only a limited number of patients. Three smaller studies, including <200 patients, confirmed the positive results of the initial study. However, all other studies, including three large multicenter studies and another study in the medical ICU by Van den Berghe's group, could not confirm the positive effects of strict blood glucose control on mortality in different cohorts of ICU patients. The largest study to date even demonstrated increased mortality in the intervention group. In addition, meta-analyses failed to show benefit in the pooled group of studies. One meta-analysis found a benefit in the subgroup of studies on surgical patients. However, a follow up meta-analysis, in which patients were classified as surgical or medical patients according to the underlying disease, and not according to the ICU in which they were admitted, could not confirm the positive effects of strict blood glucose control in the surgical cohort.

Apart from the possibility that strict blood glucose control offers no survival benefit in ICU patients, there are multiple possible explanations for the discrepancies in outcome between studies. Differences in trial design, standard of patient care, measurement of blood glucose, nutritional protocols, and patient cohorts may explain the differences in outcomes.

Hypoglycemia and glucose variability
Hypoglycemia and variation in blood glucose concentrations are two complications that may occur more frequently in a setting in which there is a less-experienced team applying the glucose protocol. Hypoglycemia in itself is a risk factor for ICU mortality. Also, several groups showed that higher blood glucose variability is associated with worse outcomes. A dedicated and well-trained team

is probably better at applying the protocol and, thus, at preventing these two complications, compared to other less well-trained or dedicated units such as those in multicenter studies. These considerations support the use of an automatic closed-loop system for blood glucose control such as currently under development.

Recommendations for blood glucose control

The current consensus guideline of the Surviving Sepsis Campaign, recommend blood glucose control <150 mg/dL. Given the risk for hypoglycemia when glucose control is in less experienced hands, some currently recommend blood glucose control between 110 and 150 mg/dL for ICU patients.

Hyperglycemic crisis and DKA or HHC

Diabetic ketoacidosis and HHC are two manifestations that may complicate hyperglycemia in diabetics. Diabetic ketoacidosis can occur in type 1 and type 2 diabetics, whereas HHC mainly occurs in type 2 diabetics. Diabetic ketoacidosis is an acute event, and may occur within a 24-hour time frame. HHC typically evolves over days to weeks. These conditions are associated with a 1 percent mortality, which may increase to 5 percent in patients >60 years of age or in patients with severe concomittant illness.

Pathogenesis

Diabetic ketoacidosis and HHC have a common pathophysiologic pathway. Increased concentrations of counterregulatory hormones such as catecholamines, cortisol, glucagon, and growth hormone, in combination with absolute or relative insulin deficiency, as in, respectively, DKA and HHC, lead to increased glucose concentrations. In DKA, there is also lipolysis, and in the liver oxidation of fatty acids to ketone bodies (β-hydroxybutyrate and acetoacetate). In both conditions, hyperglcemia is associated with a severe inflammatory reaction and procoagulant state, with increased pro-inflammatory cytokines (tumor necrosis factor-α, interleukin- β, -6, and -8), C-reactive protein, reactive oxygen species, lipid peroxidation, and plasminogen activator inhibtor-1. These return to normal within hours after adequate therapy.

Diagnosis

Diabetic ketoacidosis is characterized by increased blood glucose and metabolic acidosis caused by ketones, whereas HHC has much more pronounced hyperglyemia, dehydration, and decreased consciousness. The diagnostic criteria for both conditions are summarized in Table 18.1. Although hyperglycemia is a key diagnostic criterion, approximaly 10 percent of DKA patients present with glucose concentrations <250 mg/dL or "euglycemic DKA." This is attributed to exogenous insulin administration, food restriction, and inhibition of gluconeogenisis.

Table 18.1 **Diagnostic criteria and additional symptoms and laboratory findings for diabetic ketoacidosis (DKA) and hyperglycemic hyperosmolar coma (HHC)**

Diagnostic criteria	DKA	HHC
Blood glucose (mg/dL)	>250	>600
Arterial pH	<7.30	>7.30
Serum bicarbonate (mmol/L)	<18	>18
Ketone in urine/serum*	+	Small
Plasma osmolality mOsm/kg	Variable	>320
Anion gap	Increased	Variable
Mental status	Alert to stupor/coma	Stupor/coma

* Routine measurement of ketone bodies (e.g., on urine stick) only assesses acetoacetate and not ß-hydroxybutyrate. Therefore, these tests can underestimate the severity of ketosis.
Adapted from Kitabchi AE, Umpierrez GE, Miles JM, et al. Hyperglycemic crises in adult patients with diabetes. *Diabetes Care.* 2009;32(7): 1335–1343.

In patients with hyperglycemia and high anion gap acidosis, DKA should be differentiated from other causes for increased anion gap, such as lactic acidosis, or intoxications with, for example, salicylates, methanol, or ethylene glycol.

Symptoms and additional laboratory findings

Increased blood glucose leads to a flux of intracellular water to the extracellular compartment. Hyperglycemia will also induce osmotic diuresis, which will lead to dehydration.

Symptoms of DKA and HHC include polyuria, polydipsia, weight loss, weakness, and altered mental state. Patients have signs of dehydration such as poor skin turgor and tachycardia, tachypnea, and fever or hypothermia. Diabetic ketoacidosis patients may also have abdominal complaints, such as nausea, vomiting, and diffuse abdominal pain.

Diabetic ketoacidosis is associated with increased white blood count (WBC), even when there is no infection involved. Serum sodium concentration is decreased as a consequence of influx of water to the extracellular compartment. Pseudohyponatremia may occur when chylomicron concentrations are increased. Serum potassium is usually elevated or normal, although osmotic diuresis results in important losses of potassium. Acidemia and insulin deficiency cause a temporal loss of potassium from the intracellular compartment to the extracellular compartment. During treatment, correction of acidemia and hyperglycemia will result in a shift of potassium to the intracellular compartment and hypokalemia. Potassium levels should, therefore, be carefully followed during treatment. Similar to potassium, phosphate concentrations are usually elevated on admission. This is also a consequence of a shift from within the cell.

Although serum amylase and lipase may be elevated in DKA, this does not necesarilly indicate pancreatis.

Table 18.2 Principles of treatment of hyperglycemic crisis—diabetic ketoacidosis (DKA) or hyperglycemic hyperosmolar coma (HHC)

Treat the underlying cause—most infection

Fluid therapy	• Start, until serum Na⁺ is normal: isotonic saline
	   a. Start 15–50 mL/kg/hour
	   b. Follow up: 250–500 mL/hour, adjust to hemodynamic status and urine output
	 • Serum Na⁺ is normal: NaCl 0.45%, 250–500 mL/hour, adjust to hemodynamic status and urine output
	 • Blood glucose <200 mg/dL: glucose 5% + NaCl

Insulin	• With bolus:
	   • Bolus 0.1 U/kg IV
	   • Continuous IV infusion, start at 0.1 U/kg/hour
	 • Without bolus
	   • Continuous IV infusion, start at 0.14 U/kg/hour
	 • Titrate so that blood glucose decline is 50–75 mg/dL/hour
	 • Decrease rate to 0.02–0.05 U/kg/hour
	   • DKA: when blood glucose <200 mg/dL
	   • HHC: when blood glucose <300 mg/dL
	 • Subcutaneous route of administration:
	   • When food by mouth
	   • When DKA or HHC is resolved

Potassium	• When serum potassium < upper normal limit: 20–30 mmol per L of fluid replacement
Bicarbonate	• When blood pH<6.90: 100 mmol added to 400 mL sterile water, IV at 200 mL/h for 2 hours, until pH>7.20.

Adapted from Kitabchi AE, Umpierrez GE, Miles JM, et al. Hyperglycemic crises in adult patients with diabetes. *Diabetes Care.* 2009;32(7): 1335–1343.

Precipitating event

The most common precipitating event leading to DKA and HHC is acute disease, most often an infection. Diabetic ketoacidosis is also a common presenting symptom of new onset DM, both type 1 and type 2, or it may occur in patients with weak compliance for insulin therapy. Pregnant women who have DM may develope DKA at lower glucose elevations.

Therapy

The therapy of DKA and HHC is similar and involves correction of fluid depletion and hyperglycemia (outlined in Table 18.2). Typically, hyperglycemia is corrected faster than ketoacidosis. Therefore, after correction of glucose, insulin treatment needs to be prolonged. This means that, at this stage of therapy, glucose solutions should be administered to prevent development of hypoglycemia.

Table 18.3 Criteria for resolution of DKA or HHC
• Blood glucose <200 mg/dL
• For HHC: normalization of serum osmol and mental state
• And two of the following:
• Bicarbonate >15 mmol/L
• pH>7.30
• Anion gap≤12 mEq/L

Kitabchi AE, Umpierrez GE, Miles JM, et al. Hyperglycemic crises in adult patients with diabetes. *Diabetes Care.* 2009;32(7): 1335–1343.

Treatment of DKA and HHC is a dynamic enterprise, and it should be very carefully monitored. Blood pH and glucose are initially typically monitored every 30 minutes to every hour.

In addition to fluid and insulin, therapy should also consist of treatment of the precipitating cause of DKA or HHC.

Fluid therapy

The goal is to restore fluid deficits within a 24-hour treatment period. Aggressive fluid loading is, therefore, necessary. Initial fluid therapy consists of administration of isotonic saline infused at a rate of 15–50 mL/kg body weight per hour. Subsequent fluid therapy depends on clincial parameters such as urine output and hemodynamic status. Frequent clinical evaluations should prevent development of fluid overload and pulmonary edema. Generally, NaCl 0.45 percent is infused at 250–500 mL/h. If sodium levels are low, isotonic saline is continued.

When blood glucose concentrations are <200 mg/dL, glucose 5 percent solutions should be used for fluid replacement.

Insulin

Administration of insulin is the mainstay of treatment in DKA. Intravenous (IV) administration is the prefered route, because of the short half-live and easy titration, without delayed onset or prolonged half-life. However, also intramuscular and subcutaneous administration of insulin was effective in treating DKA.

Classicaly, insulin is started with an IV bolus of regular insuline of 0.1 units (U)/kg body weight, followed by a continuous infusion at a rate of 0.1 U/kg/h. Alternatively, you can also start with a continuous infusion, without bolus, at a rate of 0.14 U/kg/h. The rate of insulin adminsitration should be titrated to a 50–75 mg/dL/h decline of blood glucose until a steady decline is achieved. The rate of insulin should be decreased when blood glucose is <200 mg/dL in DKA and <300 mg/dL HHC to 0.02–0.05 U/kg/h. A combination of insulin and glucose 5 percent solution should be continued untill HHC or DKA are resolved.

Patients can be transitioned to subcutaneous insulin when DKA or HHC is resolved and patients start eating by mouth.

Criteria for resolution of DKA and HHC are blood glucose <200 mg/dL, and two of the following criteria are met: serum bicarbonate >15 mmol/L, venous pH>7.3, and anion gap ≤ 12 mEq/L. For HHC, serum osmolality and mental state should also be normalized (Table 18.3).

Correction of electrolytes

Potassium

Total body potassium is depleted, whereas serum concentrations in most patients are normal or high normal. Correction of acidemia and administration of insulin can result in a shift of potassium to intracellular and hypokalemia. Therefore, potassium suppletion should start when serum potassium falls below the upper normal limit. Typically, 20–30 mmol of potassium is added to each liter of replacement fluid.

When DKA patients' present with hypokalemia, initiation of insulin therapy should only begin after correction of serum potassium, in order to prevent life-threatening cardiac arrhythmias.

Bicarbonate

Severe acidosis may have diverse effects such as decreased myocardial contractility, cerebral vasodilatation and coma, and gastrointestinal complications. Despite this, bicarbonate therapy in DKA is controversial. In patients with pH between 6.9 and 7.1, studies could not demonstrate a benefit of bicarbonate therapy. There are possible deleterious effects such as hypokalemia, cerebral edema, paradoxical central nervous system acidosis, and decreased tissue oxygen uptake. There are no studies in patients with pH<6.90. Because the benefits of correcting acidosis with bicarbonate in these severly acidotic patients probably are greater than the side effects of bicarbonate, the guidelines by the American Diabetes Association (ADA) recommends administration of bicarbonate when pH<6.9. Bicarbonate (100 mmol added to 400 mL sterile water) should in these patients be administered IV at a rate of 200 mL/h for 2 hours until the venous pH>7.2.

Phosphate

Whole-body phosphate stores are decreased, however, serum phosphate is generally normal or increased in patients with DKA or HHC. During therapy, serum phospate will go intracellular, and serum phosphate may decrease. This, in turn, may result in depression of skeletal, respiratory, and cardiac muscle function. However, studies could not demonstrate a benefit of phosphate supplementation. An untoward effect of phosphate administration may be hypocalcemia.

Metformin associated with lactic acidosis

The biguanide metformin is frequently used in type 2 diabetics with concommittant obesity.

Biguanides interfere with gluconeogenesis from pyruvate and lactic acid, and can thereby result in accumulation of lactate, especially in patients with decreased kidney function because metformin is cleared by the kidneys. An earlier biguanide, phenformin, was withdrawn because of association with lactic acidosis.

The data on an association of metformin and lactic acidosis are less clear. A Cochrane systematic review on 347 studies, including 96,295 patients, could not identify a case of fatal or nonfatal lactic acidosis. The maximum incidence in patients exposed to metformin was comparable to that of control patients (4 versus 5 cases per 100,000 patients per year).

These data suggest that lactic acidosis is associated with underlying co-morbidity and not with metformin use.

Therapy for metformin associated lactic acidosis consists of supportive care. In addition, intermittent hemodialysis or continuous venovenous hemofiltration can be used to correct acid-base status and eliminate lactate and metformin.

Suggested readings

Ahmad R, Cherry RA, Lendel I, et al. Increased hospital morbidity among trauma patients with diabetes mellitus compared with age- and injury severity score-matched control subjects. *Arch Surg.* 2007;*142*(7):613–618.

Ali NA, O'Brien JMJ, Dungan K, et al. Glucose variability and mortality in patients with sepsis. *Crit Care Med.* 2008;*36*(8): 2316–2321.

Bagshaw SM, Bellomo R, Jacka MJ, et al. The impact of early hypoglycemia and blood glucose variability on outcome in critical illness. *Crit Care.* 2009;*13*(3): R91.

Bostom AD. Prevention of post-transplant cardiovascular disease—report and recommendations of an ad hoc group. *Am J Transplant.* 2002 Jul;*2*(6):491–500. PubMed PMID: 12118892.

Brunkhorst FM, Engel C, Bloos F, et al. Intensive insulin therapy and pentastarch resuscitation in severe sepsis. *N Engl J Med.* 2008;*358*(2):125–139.

Center for Disease Control and Prevention (2007) National Diabetes Fact Sheet, 2007:1–14.

Cheung NW, Wong VW, McLean M. (2006) The hyperglycemia: Intensive insulin infusion in infarction (HI-5) study: A randomized controlled trial of insulin infusion therapy for myocardial infarction. *Diabetes Care.* 2006;*29*(4): 765–770.

DeFronzo, RA. *International Textbook of Diabetes Mellitus.* 3rd ed. Chichester, West Sussex. Hoboken, NJ: Wiley; 2004.

Dellinger RP, Levy MM, Carlet JM, et al. Surviving Sepsis Campaign: International guidelines for management of severe sepsis and septic shock: 2008. *Crit Care Med.* 2008;*36*(1): 296–327.

Egi M, Bellomo R, Stachowski E, et al. Blood glucose concentration and outcome of critical illness: the impact of diabetes. *Crit Care Med.* 2008;*36*(8):2249–2255.

Falciglia M, Freyberg RW, Almenoff PL, et al. Hyperglycemia-related mortality in critically ill patients varies with admission diagnosis. *Crit Care Med.* 2009;*37*(12): 3001–3009.

Finfer S, Chittock DR, Su SY, et al. Intensive versus conventional glucose control in criti-cally ill patients. *N Engl J Med*. 2009;*360*(13):1283–1297.

Fisher JN, Shahshahani MN, Kitabchi AE. Diabetic ketoacidosis: Low-dose insulin therapy by various routes. *N Engl J Med*.1977;*297*(5):238–241.

Fishman JA. Infection in renal transplant recipients. *Semin Nephrol*. 2007 Jul;*27*(4):445–461. Review. PubMed PMID: 17616276.

Friedman GS. Hypercoagulable states in renal transplant candidates: impact of antico-agulation upon incidence of renal allograft thrombosis. *Transplantation*. 2001 Sep 27;*72*(6):1073–1078. PubMed PMID: 11579303.

Friedrich JO, Chant C, Adhikari NK. Does intensive insulin therapy really reduce mortality in critically ill surgical patients? A reanalysis of meta-analytic data. *Crit Care*. 2010;*14*(5): 324.

Gamba G, Oseguera J, Castrejon M, et al. Bicarbonate therapy in severe diabetic ketoacidosis. A double blind, randomized, placebo controlled trial. *Rev Invest Clin*. 1991;*43*(3):234–238.

Griesdale DE, de Souza RJ, van Dam RM, et al. Intensive insulin therapy and mortality among critically ill patients: a meta-analysis including NICE-SUGAR study data. *CMAJ*. 2009;*180*(8): 821–827.

Hermanides J, Bosman RJ, Vriesendorp TM. Hypoglycemia is associated with intensive care unit mortality. *Crit Care Med*. 2010;*38*(6):1430–1434.

Hermanides J, Engstrom AE, Wentholt IM, et al. Sensor-augmented insulin pump ther-apy to treat hyperglycemia at the coronary care unit: A randomized clinical pilot trial. *Diabetes Technol Ther*. 2010;*12*(7):537–542.

Hermanides J, Vriesendorp TM, Bosman RJ, et al. Glucose variability is associated with intensive care unit mortality. *Crit Care Med*. 2010;*38*(3):838–842.

Issa N. Pulmonary hypertension is associated with reduced patient survival after kidney transplantation. *Transplantation*. 2008 Nov 27;*86*(10):1384–1388. PubMed PMID: 19034007.

Kitabchi AE, Murphy MB, Spencer J, et al. Is a priming dose of insulin necessary in a low-dose insulin protocol for the treatment of diabetic ketoacidosis? *Diabetes Care*. 2008;*31*(11):2081–2085.

Kitabchi AE, Umpierrez GE, Miles JM, et al. Hyperglycemic crises in adult patients with diabetes. *Diabetes Care*. 2009;*32*(7): 1335–1343.

Kolman L, Hu YC, Montgomery DG, et al. Prognostic value of admission fasting glucose levels in patients with acute coronary syndrome. *Am J Cardiol*. 2009;*104*(4):470–474.

Malone ML, Gennis V, Goodwin JS. Characteristics of diabetic ketoacidosis in older versus younger adults. *J Am Geriatr Soc*. 1992;*40*(11):1100–1104.

Marik PE, Preiser JC. Toward understanding tight glycemic control in the ICU: A system-atic review and metaanalysis. *Chest*. 2010;*137*(3): 544–551.

Meyfroidt G, Keenan DM, Wang X, et al. Dynamic characteristics of blood glucose time series during the course of critical illness: Effects of intensive insulin therapy and relative association with mortality. *Crit Care Med*. 2010;*38*(4):1021–1029.

Morris LR, Murphy MB, Kitabchi AE. Bicarbonate therapy in severe diabetic ketoacidosis. *Ann Intern Med*. 1986;*105*(6):836–840.

Nair S, Yadav D, Pitchumoni CS. Association of diabetic ketoacidosis and acute pan-creatitis: observations in 100 consecutive episodes of DKA. *Am J Gastroenterol*. 2000;*95*(10):2795–2800.

Peters N, Jay N, Barraud D, et al. Metformin-associated lactic acidosis in an intensive care unit. *Crit Care.* 2008;*12*(6): R149.

Pfeffer MA; TREAT Investigators. A trial of darbepoetin alfa in type 2 diabetes and chronic kidney disease. *N Engl J Med.* 2009 Nov 19;*361*(21):2019–2032. PubMed PMID: 19880844.

Preiser JC, Devos P, Ruiz-Santana S, et al. A prospective randomised multi-centre controlled trial on tight glucose control by intensive insulin therapy in adult intensive care units: the Glucontrol study. *Intensive Care Med.* 2009;*35*(10):1738–1748.

Ramakrishna G, Sprung J, Ravi BS, et al. Impact of pulmonary hypertension on the outcomes of noncardiac surgery: predictors of perioperative morbidity and mortality. *J Am Coll Cardiol.* 2005 May 17;*45*(10):1691–1699. PubMed PMID: 15893189.

Ryden L, Standl E, Bartnik M, et al. Guidelines on diabetes, pre-diabetes, and cardiovascular diseases: executive summary. The Task Force on Diabetes and Cardiovascular Diseases of the European Society of Cardiology (ESC) and of the European Association for the Study of Diabetes (EASD). *Eur Heart J.* 2007;*28*(1):88–136.

Salpeter SR, Greyber E, Pasternak GA, et al. Risk of fatal and nonfatal lactic acidosis with metformin use in type 2 diabetes mellitus. *Cochrane Database Syst Rev.* 2010;(4): CD002967.

Schnell O, Schafer O, Kleybrink S, et al. Intensification of therapeutic approaches reduces mortality in diabetic patients with acute myocardial infarction: the Munich registry. *Diabetes Care.* 2004;*27*(2):455–460.

Shaheen MF, Impact of recipient and donor nonimmunologic factors on the outcome of deceased donor kidney transplantation. *Transplant Proc.* 2010 Jan-Feb;*42*(1):273–276. PubMed PMID: 20172328.

Sinnaeve PR, Steg PG, Fox KA, et al. Association of elevated fasting glucose with increased short-term and 6-month mortality in ST-segment elevation and non-ST-segment elevation acute coronary syndromes: the Global Registry of Acute Coronary Events. *Arch Intern Med.* 2009;*169*(4):402–409.

Stegenga ME, Vincent JL, Vail GM, et al. Diabetes does not alter mortality or hemostatic and inflammatory responses in patients with severe sepsis. *Crit Care Med.* 2010;*38*(2): 539–545.

Umpierrez GE, Cuervo R, Karabell A. Treatment of diabetic ketoacidosis with subcutaneous insulin aspart. *Diabetes Care.* 2004;*27*(8):1873–1878.

Umpierrez GE, Latif K, Stoever J. Efficacy of subcutaneous insulin lispro versus continuous intravenous regular insulin for the treatment of patients with diabetic ketoacidosis. *Am J Med.* 2004;*117*(5):291–296.

Van den Berghe G, Wilmer A, Hermans G, et al. Intensive insulin therapy in the medical ICU. *N Engl J Med.* 2006;*354*(5):449–461.

Van den Berghe G, Wouters PJ, Bouillon R, et al. Outcome benefit of intensive insulin therapy in the critically ill: Insulin dose versus glycemic control. *Crit Care Med.* 2003;*31*(2): 359–366.

Van den Berghe G, Wouters P, Weekers F, et al. *Intensive insulin therapy in critically ill patients. N Engl J Med.* 2001;*345*(19):1359–1367.

Vardakas KZ, Siempos II, Falagas ME. (2007) Diabetes mellitus as a risk factor for nosocomial pneumonia and associated mortality. *Diabet Med.* 2007;*24*(10):1168–1171.

Viallon A, Zeni F, Lafond P, et al. (1999) Does bicarbonate therapy improve the management of severe diabetic ketoacidosis? *Crit Care Med.* 1999;*27*(12):2690–2693.

Vincent JL. Blood glucose control in 2010: 110 to 150 mg/dL and minimal variability. *Crit Care Med.* 2010;*38*(3): 993–995.

Vincent J-L, Preiser J-C, Sprung C, et al. Insulin-treated diabetes is not associated with increased mortality in critically ill patients. *Critical Care.* 2010;*14*(1):R12.

Wang JH, Kasiske BL. Screening and management of pretransplant cardiovascular disease. *Curr Opin Nephrol Hypertens.* 2010 Nov;*19*(6):586–591. PubMed PMID: 20948378

Wasmuth HE, Kunz D, Graf J, et al. Hyperglycemia at admission to the intensive care unit is associated with elevated serum concentrations of interleukin-6 and reduced ex vivo secretion of tumor necrosis factor-??*. *Crit Care Med.* 2004;*32*(5):1109–1114.

Whitcomb BW, Pradhan EK, Pittas AG, et al. Impact of admission hyperglycemia on hospital mortality in various intensive care unit populations. *Crit Care Med.* 2005;*33*(12):2772–2777.

Wiener RS, Wiener DC, Larson RJ. Benefits and risks of tight glucose control in critically ill adults: a meta-analysis. *JAMA.* 2008;*300*(8):933–944.

Chapter 19

Thyroid conditions in critical care

James Desemone

Thyroid conditions are common in the general population and consequently are frequently found in patients admitted to the ICU. Under normal conditions, the thyroid gland primarily secretes T4 (levothyroxine) and to a lesser extent T3 (liothyronine). T3, which is regarded as the active hormone for the nuclear membrane-based thyroid receptor, can also be produced in target tissues under the regulation of local deiodinase enzymes. Entrapment and organification of iodine, as well as the synthesis and release of thyroid hormone, are under the control of the anterior pituitary hormone TSH (thyroid stimulating hormone), which, in turn, is controlled by the release of thyrotropin releasing hormone (TRH) from the hypothalamus.

Preexisting hypothyroidism

The prevalence of thyroid deficiency increases with age, and in adults over the age of 60 in the Framingham study the prevalence of thyroid deficiency was 4.4 percent overall. The prevalence in women was 5.9 percent and in men was 2.3 percent. With such a high prevalence, it is not surprising that patients with hypothyroidism are frequently admitted to the ICU, though it is rare that the primary reason for admission to the ICU is to treat the thyroid illness. In the United States, the most common cause of hypothyroidism is autoimmune (Hashimoto's) thyroiditis. Worldwide the most common cause of hypothyroidism is iodine deficiency. Other causes of hypothyroidism include surgery and I-131 radioablative therapy, both of which are treatment options for hyperthyroidism from Graves disease or multinodular goiter.

Oral thyroid hormone replacement requirements in patients with hypothyroidism do not change significantly when they are admitted to a critical care unit. If the patient's daily oral dose of levothyroxine has been stable for more than 3–4 months, that dose may be continued if the patient is able to swallow safely. If the patient is unable to swallow or there is a risk of aspiration, consideration should be given to administering levothyroxine parenterally. There is no intramuscular preparation of levothyroxine, but it may be administered intravenously.

Intravenous administration is generally tolerated well, and because 80 percent of an orally administered dose is absorbed, the dose of IV thyroid hormone should be somewhat less than the corresponding oral dose. Frequently a dose about 50 percent of the oral dose is chosen. Because the half-life of T4 is one week, missing one or two days of thyroid replacement is not critical. Thyroid replacement therapy with liothyronine (T3), which has a half-life of 1 day, is not necessary because the physiologic conversion of T4 to T3 occurs at the tissue level and is controlled by deiodinase enzymes. Both T4 and T3 are metabolized in the liver by the CYP450 system.

IV dose = ~50 percent of oral dose.

Preexisting and newly diagnosed hyperthyroidism

In the general population, hyperthyroidism is about 5–10 times less common than hypothyroidism. The prevalence of hyperthyroidism, which frequently is subclinical and increases with age, is estimated to be between 0.05 percent and 1.3 percent. The most common causes are autoimmune Graves disease, in which autoantibodies stimulate the TSH receptor on thyrocytes, and toxic uninodular and multinodular goiter.

Definitive treatment for hyperthyroidism usually involves surgery (total thyroidectomy) or radioablative therapy with I-131. Prior to definitive treatment, the mainstay of treatment for patients with hyperthyroidism is the use of one of the thionamides, propylthiouracil (PTU) or methimazole, given orally daily. These medications inhibit the synthesis and release of thyroid hormone and inhibit the conversion of T4 to T3. When a patient becomes critically ill, either of these medications should continue at the same dose. It is a therapeutic challenge when the gastrointestinal tract is compromised, however, because in most countries, PTU and methimazole are only available in an oral form and are not routinely prepared for parenteral or rectal administration.

When this is the case, treatment options are not only directed toward the inhibition of the synthesis and release of thyroid hormone but also to reduce its effects on target tissues. Alternatives to these medications include supersaturated potassium iodide (SSKI) solution, which is administered sublingually and can provide a temporary treatment for days by blocking the release of thyroid hormone. The adrenergic effects of hyperthyroidism can be inhibited by the use of intravenous beta-blockers. The conversion of T4 to T3 can be reduced by the use of high-dose intravenous glucocorticoids.

Thyroid storm

Thyroid storm is a rare life-threatening medical emergency with a mortality rate of greater than 50 percent. It is characterized by fever, tachycardia (greater than

140 beats/min), agitation, and delirium or psychosis. It can proceed to stupor or coma. The initial intervention is the administration of PTU or methimazole via nasogastric tube. PTU is preferred because it is more effective at inhibiting T4 to T3 conversion. After waiting at least 30 minutes, sublingual administration of SSKI can be given. At any time during the course of treatment, intravenous beta-adrenergic blockade and glucocorticoids should be given.

Myxedema coma

Myxedema coma is an extreme form of hypothyroidism, with about 300 cases reported in the literature. It was first described in the late 1800s, and now is rare because of improvements in detection and treatment of hypothyroidism. Nonetheless, it is important to diagnose myxedema coma since even with treatment, the mortality rate is nearly 60 percent. Since hypothyroidism is up to 8 times more common in women than men, and the prevalence of hypothyroidism increases with age, elderly women are at the highest risk for this condition. There usually is a history of surgical or autoimmune hypothyroidism, usually associated with nonadherence to thyroid replacement therapy, in which lack of feedback to the pituitary and hypothalamus leads to elevated TSH levels and occasionally to pituitary enlargement from hyperplasia. Primary hypothalamic or pituitary diseases cause fewer than 5 percent of the cases of myxedema coma and are characterized by a low, usually undetectable, TSH level. In these cases, diagnostic possibilities include Sheehan's Syndrome and infiltrating neoplastic, infectious or inflammatory conditions of the hypothalamus or pituitary.

Factors that are associated with, or can precipitate, myxedema coma include:

Hypothermia.
Cerebrovascular accidents.
Cardiomegaly.
Bradycardia.
Decreased intravascular volume.
Cardiovascular collapse.
Infections.
Anesthetics.
Sedatives.
Tranquilizers.
Narcotics.
Amiodarone.
Lithium carbonate.
Trauma.
Hypoglycemia.
Hyponatremia.
Hypoxemia.
Hypercapnia.

Treatment of myxedema coma should first address hypotension, hypothermia, and hypoventilation. Due to the high association of myxedema coma and primary or secondary adrenal insufficiency, the hypothalamic-pituitary-adrenal (HPA) axis should be evaluated and glucocorticoid replacement with intravenous hydrocortisone should be started immediately. If this is not done, initiation of thyroid replacement therapy could increase the clearance of endogenous cortisol, exacerbate underlying adrenocortical insufficiency, and precipitate Addisonian crisis. Subsequently, if the HPA axis is found to be functioning normally, hydrocortisone replacement can be discontinued.

For patients with myxedema coma, thyroid replacement is life saving. Debates regarding whether to use T4 or T3 at initiation of treatment have been raised. T4 has a longer half-life(~1 week) which makes it more reliable to monitor with serum measurements. Its drawback is that it depends on tissue conversion of T4 to T3 for activation, and this may be encumbered by inhibition of deiodinase enzymes due to the severity of the hypothyroid state. T3 has a shorter half-life (~1 day) and does not require activation, but its administration would result in nonphysiologic rises and falls in T3 levels and be difficult to monitor with serum level measurements.

Treatment is somewhat empiric, and the approach is guided by the desire to give a loading dose to immediately replace the total-body deficit in thyroid hormone, followed by administering a daily maintenance dose. Therefore, it is recommended to administer T4 200–600 mcg intravenously followed by 50–100 mcg intravenously daily until the patient is able to take the hormone enterally. If a more rapid response to thyroid replacement is needed, T3 replacement therapy may also be given for the first 2–3 days of therapy at a dose of 10 mcg intravenously every 8–12 hours. At that point, the maintenance dose of T4 should suffice. Using T3 may increase the risk of cardiovascular side effects.

Nonthyroidal illness syndrome (NTIS)

Nonthyroidal illness syndrome is seen in up to 70 percent of critically ill patients and is thought to be an adaptive response of the hypothalamic-pituitary-thyroid axis to a less catabolic state. Nonthyroidal illness syndrome is frequently diagnosed by finding low serum levels of TSH, free T4, and total T3. Early changes in NTIS include decreased conversion of T4 to T3 and increased production of reverse T3 (rT3). As the severity of illness progresses, hypothalamic release of thyrotropin releasing hormone (TRH) and pituitary release of TSH decrease, both of which contribute to lower T4 levels. Despite a low T4 level, the TSH may be in the normal laboratory reference range or lower, mimicking central hypothyroidism. Results from prior thyroid hormone testing can help differentiate NTIS from pre-existing primary or secondary hypothyroidism. Patients with NTIS are frequently treated with medications that may interfere with thyroid hormone release, serum protein binding or conversion of T4 to T3. Such medications include glucocorticoids, dopamine, amiodarone, beta-adrenergic blockers, phenytoin, furosemide and salicylates.

Because NTIS is considered an adaptive response, thyroid hormone replacement is not recommended. In fact, thyroid hormone supplementation in patients with NTIS may increase morbidity and mortality, and in patients with advanced heart failure or renal failure, it can be especially dangerous.

Suggested readings

Adler SM, Wartofsky L. The non-thyroidal illness syndrome. *Endocrinol Metab Clin N Am.* 2007;36(3):657–667.

Alfadhli E, Gianoukakis AG. Management of severe thyrotoxicosis when the gastrointestinal tract is compromised. *Thyroid.* 2011;21(3):215–220.

Sawin CT, et al. The aging thyroid: thyroid deficiency in the Framingham Study. *Arch Intern Med.* 1985;145:1386–1388.

Tietgens ST, Leinung MC. Thyroid storm. *Med Clin North Am.* 1995;79(1):169–184.

Wartofsky L. Myxedema coma. *Endocrinol Metab Clin N Am.* 2006;35:687–698.

Chapter 20

Adrenal disease in critical care

Abhinetri Pandula and James Desemone

The adrenal glands are located above the superior poles of both kidneys and weigh about 4 grams each. The adrenal gland is composed of the cortex and medulla. The cortex is divided into three layers: zona glomerulosa is the outermost superficial cortical layer and it releases mineralocorticoids including aldosterone. The middle layer, the zona fasciculata, releases glucocorticoids including cortisol, and the deepest cortical layer, the zona reticularis, releases androgens. Although mineralocorticoids like aldosterone have important roles in maintaining fluid and electrolyte balance, the glucocorticoids such as cortisol maintain blood glucose concentration, regulate the fat and protein metabolism, and mediate the inflammatory response. The adrenal medulla is the core of the adrenal gland and it releases norepinephrine and epinephrine in response to a sympathetic stimulation. The adrenal gland has an essential role in maintaining homeostasis during periods of physical and metabolic stress.

Adrenal insufficiency

Adrenal insufficiency is very rarely seen in the general population, as its prevalence is estimated to be less than 0.01 percent. It seems to be more common in critically ill patients as approximately 28 percent of critically ill patients may have relative adrenal insufficiency (RAI). Adrenal insufficiency is termed as primary when the adrenal gland itself fails to secrete the necessary hormones. Adrenal insufficiency is considered secondary when either the pituitary fails to secrete ACTH (adrenocorticotropin hormone) or tertiary when the hypothalamus fails to secrete CRH (corticotrophin releasing hormone). Figure 20.1 illustrates the hypothalamic-pituitary-adrenal axis (HPA).

Primary adrenal insufficiency

Primary adrenal insufficiency or Addison's disease can be caused by adrenal cortical atrophy, tuberculous destruction of adrenal glands, or cancerous invasion of adrenal glands. These patients present with symptoms, signs, and laboratory findings that suggest a lack of aldosterone and cortisol. These include dizziness, syncope, and nonspecific symptoms such as nausea and vomiting, with

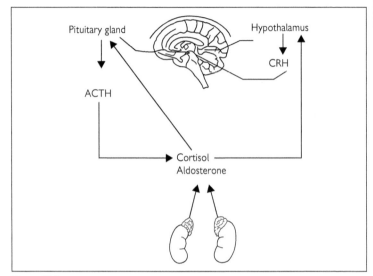

Figure 20.1

hyperkalemia, hyponatremia, hypotension, and hypoglycemia. There is an excess of ACTH in these patients because the pituitary gland and hypothalamus do not receive feedback from the impaired adrenal gland. ACTH shares a significant degree of amino acid sequence homology with melanocyte stimulating hormone (MSH) and, therefore, can stimulate melanin formation in melanocytes in the skin. Consequently, these individuals frequently present with hyperpigmentation.

Patients with primary adrenal insufficiency also present with low aldosterone levels with correspondingly elevated renin levels. Renin release from the juxta-glomerular apparatus of the kidney is stimulated by low blood pressure and low sodium and chloride concentrations in the glomerular filtrate.

Acute adrenal crisis

In acute adrenal crisis, patients present with cardiovascular collapse (shock), cyanosis, nausea, vomiting, and confusion. Though rare itself, an important cause of acute adrenal crisis is acute hemorrhagic destruction of adrenal glands (Waterhouse–Friderichsen syndrome), which can occur in previously well individuals. In children, it is typically associated with septicemia secondary to pseudomonal, meningococcal or other infections. Patients with acute adrenal hemorrhage present with abdominal, thoracic, or flank pain along with cardio-vascular collapse and fever. Acute adrenal crisis is a life-threatening emergency.

Relative adrenal insufficiency

The concept of RAI and the use of glucocorticoids in critical care patients has been investigated for over 40 years. The use of corticosteroids in these patients is controversial. Complete adrenal failure in the setting of critical illness or sepsis is rare, but under extreme stress or critical illness, the activation of the HPA axis, though present, may be suboptimal. Certain drugs such as ketoconazole and etomidate, which interfere with cortisol synthesis, and phenytoin, which increases the hepatic clearance of cortisol, can cause RAI.

Diagnosis

Primary adrenal insufficiency can usually be diagnosed with a high-dose ACTH stimulation test. Blood cortisol and ACTH levels are measured prior to administration of synthetic ACTH (cosyntropin, 250 mcg IV or IM), followed by one or two cortisol measurements within 60 minutes. Patients with primary adrenal insufficiency have high baseline ACTH levels and little or no increase in cortisol after ACTH administration. Low aldosterone and high renin levels are also found in these patients.

In critically ill patients, a random serum cortisol may be checked. Most clinicians believe that a random cortisol of less than 15 mcg/dl during critical illness and failure to observe an increase in cortisol of 9 mcg/dl or greater after a high-dose ACTH stimulation test is indicative of relative adrenal insufficiency. An increase in serum cortisol after stimulation with cosyntropin that is less than 9 mcg/dl is associated with increased mortality in septic shock.

A more sensitive test to detect relative adrenal insufficiency is the low-dose (1 mcg IM or IV) ACTH stimulation test.

Treatment

Treatment involves replacing the hormones that the adrenal glands are lacking. Cortisol can be replaced with a synthetic glucocorticoids such as hydrocortisone, prednisone, methylprednisolone, dexamethasone, taken orally once to three times each day. Nonstressed daily production of cortisol in adults is 15–25 mg/day, and the maximum stressed cortisol production is between 200 to 350 mg/day. Thus, a daily dose of hydrocortisone 25–200 mg/day is considered low dose, 200–350 mg/day is a physiological stress dose, 351–1000 mg/day is a supra-physiological stress dose. In patients with primary adrenal insufficiency aldosterone deficiency may be treated with enteral fludrocortisone acetate (Florinef), taken once or twice a day.

Complications associated with the long-term use of high-dose corticosteroids include immune suppression, increased risk of infection, impaired wound healing, hyperglycemia, steroid induced myopathy, suppression of HPA axis, and psychosis.

Secondary adrenal insufficiency

Secondary adrenal insufficiency occurs due to lack of ACTH. In this form of adrenal insufficiency, aldosterone is not affected. One of the most common causes of secondary adrenal insufficiency is the long-term use of exogenous glucocorticoids given for the treatment of nonendocrine diseases such as rheumatoid disease, inflammatory bowel disease, or chronic obstructive pulmonary disease. Other causes of secondary adrenal insufficiency are surgery, infarction, tumors, and infiltrative diseases involving the pituitary gland.

Acute adrenal crisis can be precipitated by rapid withdrawal from glucocorticoids in patients who have been chronically treated with these medications.

Hypercortisolism—Cushing's syndrome

Cushing's syndrome is a disease complex that is caused by prolonged exposure of body organs to elevated levels of serum cortisol. Cushing's syndrome is rare and generally affects people between ages of 20 to 50. It can be caused by primary or ectopic production of cortisol from benign or malignant tumors, as well as ectopic production of ACTH from benign or malignant tumors. Chronic use of glucocorticoids for autoimmune disorders such as rheumatoid arthritis or lupus, or for treatment of COPD and asthma can cause iatrogenic Cushing's syndrome.

Benign ACTH-secreting pituitary adenomas can secrete large amounts of ACTH, and this, in turn, causes adrenal hyperplasia and stimulates excess secretion of cortisol. When Cushing's syndrome is caused by excess release of ACTH from the pituitary gland, the condition is named Cushing's disease. Ectopic ACTH can also be produced from tumors outside the pituitary gland. Small cell lung cancer accounts for up to 13 percent of lung cancers, and these tumors, as well as carcinoid tumors of the lung or gut, may secrete ACTH. Less commonly, thymomas, pancreatic islet cell tumors, and medullary carcinoma of the thyroid can produce ACTH. Adrenal adenomas are also more common in women, and they, too, can produce excess cortisol or ACTH.

Rare causes of Cushing's syndrome include micronodular dysplasia of the adrenals (familial Cushing's syndrome) and multiple endocrine neoplasia type 1 (MEN 1) in which patients have hormone-secreting tumors of the parathyroid, pituitary, and pancreas.

Physical findings in patients with Cushing's syndrome are rounded faces, increased fat around the neck, and slender arms and legs. Their skin is very fragile and easy to bruise. Purple to pink stretch marks may be present on the abdomen, thighs, buttocks, arms, and breasts. The excess cortisol also presents with hyperglycemia, fatigue, loss of bone density, myalgias and hypertension. Both males and females have difficulties with fertility. A fatty hump is often seen between the shoulder blades.

Diagnosis

Three tests are commonly used to diagnose Cushing's syndrome.

- The 24-hour urinary free cortisol: the normal urinary cortisol excretion rate is 10–100 micrograms per 24 hrs. A value that is 4 times above the upper limit of this range in an adult is suggestive of Cushing's syndrome.
- Overnight Dexamethasone Suppression Test: Dexamethasone 1 mg p.o. between 11:00 P.M. and 12:00 midnight, measure morning cortisol between 8:00 and 9:00 A.M. A morning serum cortisol level of <1.8 excludes Cushing's syndrome as a diagnostic possibility.

- Low dose, high dose dexamethasone suppression test: dexamethasone 0.5 mg orally every 6 hours for 2 days (low dose), followed by dexamethasone 2.0 mg orally every 6 hours for 2 days (high dose). Measure either or both the morning serum cortisol or the 24-hour urinary free cortisol. Patients with normal adrenocortical function suppress cortisol release with the low-dose test, patients with Cushing's Disease suppress with the high-dose test. Patients with Cushing's syndrome from any other cause do not suppress cortisol release with either test.

Cushing's syndrome can be confused with pseudo-Cushing's syndrome, which is seen in patients who have depression, anxiety, alcohol abuse, obesity, or polycystic ovarian syndrome. These patients frequently present with cortisol levels that are in the same range as patients with Cushing's syndrome. In these cases, more sophisticated testing using dexamethasone in combination with corticotrophin releasing hormone (CRH) stimulation testing may be required to differentiate pseudo-Cushing's syndrome from true Cushing's syndrome.

Treatment of Cushing's syndrome

Treatment of Cushing's syndrome is primarily surgical. Pituitary tumors secreting ACTH and adrenal tumors secreting cortisol or ACTH should be excised. Ectopic tumors secreting ACTH or cortisol should be localized and removed if possible. Diabetes and hypertension should be treated accordingly while the patient is awaiting surgery.

Medical treatment of Cushing's sydrome is directed to either inhibition of the enzymes of steroid synthesis (ketoconazole, metyrapone, and aminoglutethimide) or those that have an adrenolytic effect (mitotane). Of these, the antifungal medication ketoconazole is the most frequently prescribed.

Exogenous steroids should be tapered off in patients with iatrogenic Cushing's syndrome.

Primary aldosteronism—Conn syndrome

A tumor or hyperplasia of the zona glomerulosa can secrete excess aldosterone and cause hypernatremia, hypokalemia, and metabolic alkalosis in many, but not all, cases. Hypertension is a consequence of increased extracellular volume and sodium retention. Fatigue, palpitations, and headaches are common symptoms. Primary hyperaldosteronism is recognized as the cause of hypertension in 5–13 percent of patients. Some patients with primary hyperaldosteronism also have periodic muscle paralysis secondary to low extracellular potassium concentration.

Diagnosis

Primary hyperaldosteronism should be considered in patients with drug-resistant hypertension, hypokalemia, the presence of an adrenal adenoma (if found serendipitously, an "incidentaloma"), and hypertension diagnosed before the age of

20. In such patients, a morning plasma aldosterone concentration with a plasma renin activity (PRA) or a plasma renin concentration should be measured. A high aldosterone level with a low renin level is suggestive of primary hyperaldosternonism, and a ratio between the aldosterone concentration and the PRA of >20 calls for further evaluation or surgical intervention. A CT of abdomen and adrenal venous sampling may be required to clearly identify the source of excess aldosterone.

Treatment

Spironolactone can be used for the treatment of hypertension and hypokalemia as a temporary measure, but, ultimately, surgical excision of a functioning adrenal tumor or partial resection of a hyperplastic adrenal gland is usually required. Hypertension typically resolves 1–3 months after surgery.

Androgen-secreting tumors and congenital adrenal hyperplasia

Occasionally adrenocortical tumors can secrete excess androgens and cause masculinization. In female patients, this presents with hirsutism, deepening of the voice, clitoral enlargement, and development of other masculine features. In prepubertal males, the virilizing tumor causes precocious puberty with increases in bodily hair and rapid development of male secondary sex characteristics. In adult males, the androgenital syndrome is generally obscured by normal virilizing characteristics of testosterone.

Congenital adrenal hyperplasia is a heterogeneous group of disorders characterized by an absence or deficiency of one of the enzymes in the steroid biosynthetic pathway. The most severe cases present in infancy or childhood (classical), and mild cases present in adulthood (nonclassical).

The most common form of this condition is due to deficiency of the enzyme 21 hydroxylase. This deficiency leads to lower levels of cortisol, which affects the negative feedback loop to hypothalamic CRH and pituitary ACTH, and causes buildup of the precursor substrate of this enzyme, 17 hydroxyprogesterone. The elevated ACTH leads to hyperplasia of the adrenal cortices. In classical cases, salt wasting and buildup of adrenal androgens ensues. Glucocorticoid replacement in such cases is life saving.

In older patients with the milder nonclassical form, symptoms and signs are frequently subtle or unrecognized.

Diagnosis

In patients with single tumors, serum testing of testosterone, adrenal androgens, cortisol, and aldosterone levels should be considered. In patients with adrenal hyperplasia, baseline testing of cortisol, ACTH, and perhaps 17 hydroxyprogesterone should be performed. Many cases will require ACTH stimulation testing and the use of a published nomogram to clarify the diagnosis.

Treatment

Surgery is the primary treatment in patients with an adrenal tumor. The treatment for patients with congenital adrenal hyperplasia is physiologic dosing of corticosteroids.

Summary and recommendations

- Primary adrenal insufficiency is very rare in the general population, but it can be seen in up to 25 percent of critically ill patients.
- Adrenal insufficiency:
  - Primary: treated with glucocorticoids and possibly mineralocorticoids.
  - Secondary: treated with glucocorticoids alone.
- Adrenal hemorrhage is associated with cardiovascular collapse and abdominal, pelvis, flank, or thoracic pain. Fatigue, weakness, dizziness, arthralgias, nausea, and vomiting are present in up to 50 percent of these patients.
- Relative adrenal insufficiency is a controversial subject, but most agree that patients that lack adrenal reserve (less than 9 mcg/dl serum cortisol response to cosyntropin) will benefit from corticosteroid supplementation.
- Cushing's syndrome, Conn syndrome, congenital adrenal hyperplasia, and androgen secreting tumors are rarely diagnosed in a critical-care setting, but the ability to recognize them when they occur is essential to providing proper care.

Suggested readings

Guyton AC, Hall JE. *Textbook of Medical Physiology* 9th ed. Philadelphia, PA: W.B. Saunders;1996:957–970.

Kozyra EF, Wax RS, Burry LD. Can 1 mcg of cosyntropin be used to evaluate adrenal insufficiency in critically ill patients? *Ann Pharmacotherapy.* 2005;39:691–698.

Malerba G, et al. Risk factors for relative adrenocortical deficiency in intensive care patients needing mechanical ventilation. *Intens Care Med.* 2005;31:388.

Marik PE. Critical illness-related corticosteroid insufficiency. *Chest.* Jan 2009;135 (1):181–193.

Nimkam S, Lin-su K, New MI. Steroid 21 Hydroxylase deficiency congenital adrenal hyperplasia. *Endocrinol Metab Clin North Am.* 2009;38:699–718.

Oelkers W. Adrenal Insufficiency. *N Eng J Med.* 1996;335:1206–1212.

Pivonello R, et al. Cushing's syndrome. *Endocrinol Metab Clin North Am.* 2008;37:135–149.

Rivers EP. et al. Adrenal Insufficiency in high-risk surgical ICU patients. *hest.* 2001;119; 889–896

Young WF. Primary aldosteronism: renaissance of a syndrome. *Clin Endocrinol.* 2007;66:607–618.

Chapter 21

Calcium, bone, and mineral disease in the critically ill patient

Roy O. Mathew

Mineral and bone balance are frequently deranged in critically ill patients. The following discussion is meant to be a brief guide for the identification and treatment of disorders of individual ions, and maintenance of general bone health. It is always important to note, however, that the mineral and bone derangements listed here are frequently signs of an underlying disease process. Identification of a unifying diagnosis in patients with multiple presenting abnormalities will allow focused and potentially life-saving therapeutics to be initiated in a timely manner.

Calcium

Calcium plays a fundamental role in several aspects of physiology pertinent to the critical-care setting. The biologically active form is commonly measured as ionized calcium (40 percent of total plasma calcium; ~1.1 mmol/L–4.4 mg/dL). Given the poor correlation of "albumin-corrected" total calcium with ionized calcium levels, it is recommended that ionized calcium be routinely measured in high-risk populations (Vincent, 1995). Blood pH and the availability of lactate and bicarbonate in plasma (frequently abnormal in critically ill patients) will alter the ionized calcium concentration (Baker, 2002):

1. PH alterations in calcium binding by albumin.
    a. Every 0.1 unit reduction in plasma pH, the ionized calcium increases by 0.07 mmol/L.
2. Alterations in calcium complexes (typically insignificant in the clinical setting):
    a. Lactate: With every 1 mmol/L increase in lactate, the ionized calcium decreases by 0.006 mmol/L (0.02 mg/dL).
    b. Bicarbonate: With every 1 mmol/L decrease in bicarbonate there is a 0.004 mmol/L (0.02 mg/dL) increase in ionized calcium.

Hypocalcemia

The prevalence of hypocalcemia in the ICU has been reported to be up to 88% (Zivin, 2001). The presence of low calcium is often a poor prognostic sign and has been correlated with an increased incidence of sepsis, longer duration of ICU stay, and increased mortality rates. Hypocalcemia is defined as total calcium <2.1 mmol/L (8.4 mg/dL) or ionized calcium <1.15 mmol/L (4.6 mg/dL). Ionized hypocalcemia is the immediate cause of clinical symptoms. Signs and symptoms are manifest in various organ systems (Table 21.1). Classic signs of hypocalcemia include Chvostek's or Trousseau's signs: contraction of ipsilateral facial muscles by stimulation of facial nerve, spasm of arm and hand by occlusion of brachial blood supply for 3–4 minutes, respectively.

Causes

1. Associated with hyperphosphatemia:
   Renal failure.
   Rhabdomyolysis.
   Hypoparathyroidism (including surgery), pseudohypoparathyroidism.
2. Associated with low/normal phosphate:
   Critical illness including sepsis, burns.
   Hypomagnesemia.
   Pancreatitis.
   Osteomalacia.
   Overhydration.
   Massive blood transfusion (citrate-binding).
   Hyperventilation and the resulting respiratory alkalosis may reduce the ionized plasma calcium fraction and induce clinical features of hypocalcemia.

Differential diagnosis of ionized hypocalcemia in the critically ill population is broad (Table 21.2).

1. Sepsis and septic shock are associated with various inflammatory mediators that promote cellular uptake of calcium as a protective mechanism in order to reduce cellular activity.
2. In rhabdomyolysis, pancreatitis, and tumor lysis syndrome, calcium is bound and removed from the circulation: by phosphorous in rhabdomyolysis and tumor lysis syndrome, and by free fatty acids in pancreatitis.
3. Severe burn injury may have several mechanisms contributing to hypocalcemia: binding with free fatty acids, and hypoparathyroidism related to marked magnesium deficiency.
4. Volume resuscitation, with crystalloid or colloid, has been demonstrated to cause hypocalcemia.
5. Citrate anticoagulation during extracorporeal therapies or from large-volume blood-product transfusion may lead to citrate accumulation, especially in the setting of liver disease. Citrate toxicity:
   a. Elevated total calcium.
   b. Suppressed ionized calcium.
   c. Metabolic alkalosis.

Table 21.1 Clinical manifestations and suggested treatment regimens

Element	Normal range	Problem	Clinical manifestations	Treatment
Calcium	Total: 2.1–2.55 mmol/L (8.4–10.2 mg/dL) Ionized: 1.15–1.3 mmol/L (4.6–5.2 mg/dL)	Ionized hypocalcemia	1. CARDIOVASCULAR: a. Hypotension (often refractory to pressor support) b. Cardiac dysrhythmia (prolongation of QTc; premature ventricular contractions; torsade des pointes) 2. NEUROLOGIC: a. Paresthesias b. Cramps c. Mental status changes d. Chvostek's or Trousseau's signs e. Tetany	1. Ionized calcium 1- 1.15 mmol/l: a. 2 gm of calcium gluconate 2. Ionized calcium <1 mmol/l: a. 4 gm of calcium gluconate *All doses administered via central venous access, and rate is 1 gm/hr. If respiratory alkalosis is present, adjust ventilator settings or if spontaneously hyperventilating and agitated calm or sedate. Rebreathing into a bag can be beneficial. If hypotensive or with decreased cardiac output after calcium antagonist give 5–10 ml 10% calcium chloride over 2–5 minutes Correct hypomagnesesmia or hypokalemia if present
		Ionized hypercalcemia	1. CARDIOVASCULAR: a. Shortening of QT interval b. ST segment elevation mimicking acute myocardial infarction 2. NEUROMUSCULAR: a. Lethargy b. Confusion c. Stupor d. Weakness	1. Mild to moderate hypercalcemia with symptoms: Saline-diuresis (saline to maintain urine output at 100–150 ml/hr ± furosemide IV 40–60 mg every 2 to 4 hours). 2. Severe hypercalcemia (primary hyperparathyroidism, malignancy): a. Pamidronate 60–90 mg IV once over 2 hours. (30–45 mg in impaired renal function) b. Zoledronic acid (more potent and preferred in malignancy related hypercalcemia) 4 mg over 15–30 minutes IV c. Hemodialysis

Table 21.1 (continued)

Element	Normal range	Problem	Clinical manifestations	Treatment
			3. GASTROINTESTINAL: a. Constipation b. Nausea 4. RENAL: a. AKI b. Polyuria c. Hypokalaemia d. Nephrolithiasis e. Rarely type I distal tubular acidosis	
Phosphorous	0.8 to 1.35 mmol/L (2.8–4.5 mg/dL)	Hypophosphataemia	1. NEUROMUSCULAR: a. Respiratory muscle paralysis (failure to wean from ventilator) b. Spontaneous rhabdomyolysis 2. CARDIOVASCULAR: a. Hypotension, not responsive to pressor support 3. GASTROINTESTINAL: a. Ileus	14.5 mmol of phosphate IV over one hour. (As potassium salt if serum [potassium] <5 mmol/l; As the sodium salt if serum [potassium] ≥ 5 mmol/l)
		Hyperphosphataemia	1. RENAL/METABOLIC: a. Acute kidney injury if rate of rise is rapid and levels attained are high (tumor lysis, rhabdomyolysis, acute enteric phosphate toxicity) b. Hypocalcemia	1. Lowering nutritional phosphate load a. (1 gm daily or less) 2. Intestinal phosphate binders for chronic hyperphosphataemia (i.e., CKD). a. Sevelamer carbonate/Sevelamer hydrochloride (Renvela®/Renagel®, respectively) b. Lanthanum carbonate (Fosrenol®)

				3. DERMATOLOGIC: a. Calcific uremic arteriolopathy (Calciphylaxis) in severe chronic hyperphosphataemia.	3. Acute hemodialysis for severe hyperphosphataemia in tumor lysis or rhabdomyolysis. 4. Saline infusions may help with reducing phosphate levels but is associated with worsening calcium levels.
Magnesium	0.63–1 mmol/L (1.26–2 meq/L; 1.9–2.4 mg/dL)	Hypomagnesaemia	1. METABOLIC: Hypokalaemia (recalcitrant) Hypocalcemia 2. CARDIAC: Supraventricular/ventricular dysrhythmias Coronary artery spasm 3. NEUROMUSCULAR: Fasciculation Respiratory muscle weakness Convulsions Cramps	For severe hypomagnesaemia (<0.5 mmol/L) or symptomatic 1. 2 gm magnesium sulfate in 100 ml of DSW over 5 to 10 min 2. Maintenance: a. Continuous infusion of 4 to 6 grams per day. (If renal function impaired cut above dosing in half) Monitor serum magnesium levels closely to avoid overshoot Less acute situations or asymptomatic hypomagnesemia: 1–2 g Mg sulfate solution over 1–2 hrs Continuous infusion is reserve for therapeutic goals such as management of preeclampsia or cardiac arrhythmia Oral magnesium can cause laxative effect
		Hypermagnesaemia (range of magnesium associated with the symptom)	1. METABOLIC: Ionized hypocalcemia 2. NEUROMUSCULAR: Drowsiness Hyporeflexia (4–5 mmol/L) Coma Respiratory muscle (6–7 mmol/L) 3. CARDIOVASCULAR: Hypotension Sinoatrial and atrioventricular nodal blocks (3–5 mmol/L) Asystole (10–12.5 mmol/L)	1. Requires increasing the excretion of the ion: Loop diuretics + Saline. 2. If renal function severely compromised: Hemodialysis may be required. 3. Intravenous calcium chloride may mitigate cardiovascular effects: 100–200 mg elemental calcium infused over 5–10 minutes

QTc: RR interval corrected QT interval; AKI: acute kidney injury; CKD: chronic kidney disease; D5W: 5% Dextrose in water.

CHAPTER 21 **Calcium, bone, and mineral disease**

Table 21.2 Mineral disorders differential diagnosis

Element	Problem	Differential Diagnosis		
		Renal	Gastrointestinal	Other

Calcium	Hypocalcemia	1. Citrate accumulation (citrate anticoagulated CRRT)
		2. Decreased reabsorption
		a. Decreased PTH activity
		  i. Primary or secondary hypoparathyroidism.
		  ii. Pseudohypoparathyroidism
		  iii. Hypomagnesaemia
		b. Vitamin D deficiency
		3. Increased loss of calcium
		a. Renal losses (Furosemide or saline diuresis)
			1. Decreased intake
			a. Malnutrition (prolonged critical illness; pre-existing alcoholism, dementia)
			b. Vitamin D deficiency (dietary or chronic illness, e.g., CKD)
			2. Sequestration:
			a. Pancreatitis
			3. Increased loss
			a. Small bowel surgery
				1. Redistribution: Acute respiratory alkalosis (pH induced increase in albumin binding)
				2. Calcium sequestration
				a. Post-para-thyroidectomy ("hungry-bone" syndrome)
				b. Rhabdomyolysis
				c. Acute hyperphosphataemia (e.g. tumor lysis syndrome)
				d. Critical illness (sepsis, burns, toxic shock)
				e. Fluoride toxicity
				f. Oxalate poisoning
				g. Citrate accumulation from blood products

	Hypercalcemia	1. CKD (Tertiary hyperparathyroidism) 2. Recovery from acute kidney injury 3. Tubular reabsorption: a. Lithium b. Thiazides c. Familial hypocalciuric hypercalcemia	Vitamin D intoxication	1. Malignancy a. PTHrp b. Bone metastases c. Other cytokine related (e.g., IL-6) 2. Endocrine a. Paget b. Thyrotoxicosis c. Addison's disease d. Acromegaly e. Pheo- chromocytoma 3. Granulomatous disease a. Sarcoidosis b. Tuberculosis

			Redistribution

Phosphorous	Hypophosphataemia	1. Renal replacement therapy (typically CRRT).
		2. Renal losses:
		  a. Hyperparathyroidism
		  b. Renal tubular acidosis (typically proximal in association with Fanconi syndrome)
		  c. Vitamin D deficiency
		  d. Diuretics (acetazolamide)
			1. Reduced availability (inadequate supplementation)
			2. Impaired absorption (antacid use; vitamin D deficiency)
			3. Chronic alcoholism
				1. Alkalosis
				2. Treatment of diabetic ketoacidosis
				3. Re-feeding
				4. Correction of chronic hypercapnia

	Hyperphosphataemia	Acute or chronic renal failure	1. Phosphate containing laxatives/enemas 2. Vitamin D intoxication	1. Rhabdomyolysis 2. Tumor lysis syndrome

Magnesium	Hypomagnesaemia	1. Tubular mishandling
		  Post-ATN
		  Postobstruction
		  Genetic disorders (Gitelman)
		2. Medication Induced
		  Aminoglycosides
		  Amphotericin B
		  Cisplatin
		  Cetuximab
		  Diuretics (especially loop diuretics)
			1. Chronic or acute diarrheal syndromes
			2. Intestinal bypass surgeries
			3. Severe ischemic colitis
				1. Diabetes
				2. Chronic alcohol abuse

	Hypermagnesaemia	Acute GFR decline and concomitant administration of large amounts of magnesium salts Familial hypocalciuric hypercalcemia	Magnesium containing laxatives/enemas (especially with decreased GFR)	1. Acidosis 2. Spurious elevations may be seen with hemolysis

CRRT: continuous renal replacement therapy; PTH: parathyroid hormone; CKD: chronic kidney disease; IL-6: interleukin-6; PTHrp: parathyroid hormone related protein; GFR: glomerular filtration rate; ATN: acute tubular necrosis.

CHAPTER 21 **Calcium, bone, and mineral disease**

Any life-threatening manifestation of hypocalcemia should be immediately managed with calcium replacement to normalize ionized calcium values (Table 21.1). In non-life-threatening situations, cautious normalization of hypocalcemia may be undertaken; however, more aggressive determination of contributing factors should be a priority. Citrate toxicity is unique in that the treatment is to cease further administration of citrate and allow the citrate that has accumulated to be metabolized. In cases of severe life-threatening hypocalcemia due to citrate excess infusion (i.e. by mistaken CRRT circuit connections), emergent hemodialysis will remove excess citrate efficiently. In this setting, it is not uncommon to see posttherapy hypercalcemia as the metabolism of citrate releases bound calcium.

Hypercalcemia

Among all causes of hypercalcemia, hyperparathyroidism, and malignancy are the most common, accounting for greater than 90 percent of cases (Ziegler, 2001).

Symptoms of hypercalcemia usually do not become apparent until the total (ionized + unionized) plasma levels >13 mg/dL (normal range 8.5–10.5 mg/dL). Symptoms depend on the patient's age, the duration and rate of increase of plasma calcium, and the presence of concurrent medical conditions. Signs and symptoms of hypercalcemia may include:

- Nausea, vomiting, weight loss, pruritus.
- Abdominal pain, constipation, acute pancreatitis.
- Muscle weakness, fatigue, lethargy.
- Depression, mania, psychosis, drowsiness, coma.
- Polyuria, renal calculi, renal failure.
- Cardiac arrhythmias.

Hypercalcemia is defined as a total calcium level >2.55 mmol/L (10.2 mg/dL) or ionized calcium >1.30 mmol/L (5.2 mg/dL). Important causes include:

1. Hyperparathyroidism that persists following resolution of hypocalcemia (tertiary hyperparathyroidism).
2. Primary hyperparathyroidism of unclear etiology has been purported in some cases of critical-care hypercalcemia.
3. Immobilization hypercalcemia. Two important factors have been identified that increase the risk for developing immobilization hypercalcemia:
   a. Prolonged (>20 days) immobilization.
   b. Severe renal insufficiency (creatinine clearance <30 ml/min).

Management

- Identify and treat cause where possible.
- Carefully monitor hemodynamic variables, urine output, and ECG morphology with frequent estimations of plasma Ca^{2+}, PO_4^{3-}, Mg^{2+}, Na^+, and K^+.
- Intravascular volume repletion—this inhibits proximal tubular reabsorption of calcium and may lower plasma Ca^{2+} by 1–2 mg/dL. It should precede diuretics or any other therapy. Isotonic saline is typically used.

- Calciuresis—after adequate intravascular volume repletion, a forced diuresis with furosemide plus 0.9 percent saline (6–8 l/day) may be attempted.
- Steroids can be effective for hypercalcemia related to hematological cancers (lymphoma, myeloma), vitamin D overdose and sarcoidosis.
- Calcitonin has the most rapid onset of action with a nadir often reached within 12–24 hours. Its action is limited (usually does not decrease plasma Ca^{2+} by more than 2–3 mg/dL), usually short-lived and rebound hypercalcemia may occur.
- Biphosphonates (e.g., pamidronate) and IV phosphate should only be given after other measures have failed in view of their toxicity and potential complications.
- Renal replacement therapy (RRT) may be indicated particularly early on if the patient is in established oligo-anuric renal failure ± fluid overloaded.

Renal replacement therapy without calcium in the dialysis or replacement fluid are both effective therapies for hypercalcemia, although they are usually considered treatments of last resort. Renal replacement therapy may be indicated in patients with severe malignancy-associated hypercalcemia and renal failure or heart failure, in whom hydration cannot be safely administered.

The use of continuous renal replacement therapy (CRRT) or hemodialysis in patients with hypercalcemia but without renal failure may require modification of the composition of dialysis solutions. In one case report, hemodialysis with a calcium-free dialysate resulted in rapid correction of all abnormalities in a patient in whom medical therapy had failed to reverse hypercalcemia, mental status changes to hypercalcemia of malignancy (Wang, 2009). In another report, hypophosphatemia and hypercalcemia, due to primary hyperparathyroidism, were corrected utilizing hemodialysis therapy with a phosphorous-enriched standard calcium containing dialysate (Leehey, 1997).

Drug dosage

Treatment is focused on acute and chronic management of the hypercalcemia. Acute severe hypercalcemia may be treated with aggressive volume expansion with isotonic saline plus loop diuretics to aid in calcium excretion; this is obviously contingent on an intact renal system. Saline simultaneously corrects dehydration often present with chronic hypercalcemia as well as inhibiting distal tubular reabsorption of calcium. Furosemide should be added when levels are significantly elevated or symptoms are particularly problematic. If there is severe acute kidney injury or advanced chronic kidney disease (CKD), dialysis against low or even normal calcium (≤ 2.5 meq/L–1.25 mmol/L) dialysate concentration is effective in

Diuretics	Furosemide 10–40 mg IV 2–4 hours (may be increased to 80–100 mg IV every 1–2 hours)
Steroids	Hydrocortisone 100 mg qid IV or prednisolone 40–60 mg PO for 3–5 days
Pamidronate	15–60 mg slow IV bolus
Calcitonin	3–4 U/kg IV followed by 4 U/kg SC bd

removal of excess calcium. Sustained significant reductions will require IV bisphosphonate therapy; this is especially so in malignancy and immobilization related hypercalcemia. Calcitonin may be helpful in the short term. Digitalis should not be administered during hypercalcemia as cardiac arrest may develop.

Phosphate

Phosphate is an essential component of cellular activity, bone mineralization, heme-oxygen transport, and acid-base buffering.

Hypophosphataemia

Hypophosphataemia is a common and significant disorder in critically ill patients. The causes of hypophosphatemia may be related to (Table 21.2):

1. Inappropriate gastrointestinal absorption or loss,
2. Redistribution into intra-cellular compartments (e.g. refeeding syndrome), or
3. Inappropriate renal handling of the filtered load.

   Critically ill patients may have components of all of these. Clinical consequences are most notable in the respiratory and cardiovascular systems (Table 21.1). Treatment needs to focus on two aspects of phosphate homeostasis: immediate correction of severe depletion, and chronic supplementation. All patients should be provided adequate phosphate load in the enteral or parenteral feeding sources (French, 2004). If moderate to severe hypophosphatemia is present (<0.8 mmol/L–2.48 mg/dL), acute infusion regimens have been designed to effectively raise serum phosphate levels without inducing hypocalcemia or AKI (Table 21.1). In the setting of RRT induced hypophosphatemia, efforts should be aimed at supplementation rather than reduction of RRT dose.

Hyperphosphatemia

Hyperphosphatemia is defined as serum phosphate levels >1.4 mmol/L (4.5 mg/dL). Causes fall into three broad categories (Table 21.2):

1. Increased gastrointestinal intake (uncommon in critically ill patients),
2. Endogenous release,
3. Decreased urinary clearance.

Causes

There are three general circumstances, alone or in combination, in which hyperphosphatemia occurs:

1. Massive acute phosphate load (e.g. tumor lysis, rhabdomyolysis).
2. Renal failure.
3. Increase phosphate reabsorption (hypoparathyroidism, acromegaly, familial tumoral calcinosis, bisphosphonate therapy, vitamin D toxicity).

Clinical manifestations of hyperphosphatemia are uncommon unless the rate of rise is rapid or the levels are significantly elevated. Rapid marked rise in serum phosphorous levels may lead to acute hypocalcemia (secondary to the formation of calcium-phosphorous complex) with associated neurologic complications. Rapid elevation of serum phosphorous associated with bowel preparation prior to endoscopy has been demonstrated to cause severe AKI. Chronic elevations, seen most in patients with advanced CKD, are associated with ectopic ossifications; the most devastating manifestation being calciphylaxis: a debilitating disease of dermal calcific arteriolopathy that is associated with adverse outcomes.

Recently, a class of peptides called phosphatonins has been identified that are responsible, in addition to parathyroid hormone and vitamin D, for phosphate homeostasis; the best characterized is fibroblast growth factor-23 (FGF-23). (Berndt, 2005) Zhang and colleagues examined the relationship of FGF-23 levels with survival among critically ill individuals with and without acute kidney injury (AKI) (Zhang, 2011). FGF-23 was found to be significantly higher in patients with AKI than those without AKI. For patients with AKI, FGF-23 was higher in non-survivors than in survivors. Interestingly, serum phosphorous levels and FGF-23 levels were not correlated. Further research will be needed to understand the relationship between FGF-23 and phosphate homeostasis within AKI.

Treatment may be directed at reducing gastrointestinal intake, increasing urinary excretion, or extracorporeal clearance of blood. Oral phosphate binders are calcium based, or non-calcium based (polyamine complexes); aluminum based compounds are no longer used due to toxicity. Hemodialysis (as compared to peritoneal dialysis) is efficient at acutely lowering serum phosphorous levels.

Management

The approach to therapy differs in acute and chronic hyperphosphatemia. Acute severe hyperphosphatemia with symptomatic hypocalcemia can be life-threatening. The hyperphosphatemia usually resolves within 6 to 12 hours if renal function is intact. Phosphate excretion can be increased by saline infusion, although this can further reduce the serum calcium concentration by dilution. CRRT or hemodialysis is often indicated in patients with symptomatic hypocalcemia, particularly if renal function is impaired. Unlike other electrolytes, phosphate is removed more efficiently with CRRT (in hemofiltration mode) compared to hemodialysis. This is because PO_4^{3-} acts in solution as a larger molecule and is more difficult to remove with diffusion (dialysis) compared to convection (filtration) (Tan 2001). Additionally, the large intracellular distribution of phosphate requires longer dialytic treatments, such as CRRT, to allow intercompartmental equilibration.

Pseudohyperphosphatemia

Spurious hyperphosphatemia may result from interference with the analytical methods.

Causes
- Hyperglobulinemia, hyperlipidemia, hemolysis, and hyperbilirubinemia.
- Liposomal amphotericin B.

Magnesium

Magnesium is the second most abundant intracellular cation in the body. No clear hormonal regulation of magnesium has been identified.

Magnesium is primarily an intracellular ion involved in the production and utilization of energy stores and in the mediation of nerve transmission. Low plasma levels, which do not necessarily reflect either intracellular or whole body stores, may thus be associated with features related to these functions:
- Confusion, irritability.
- Seizures.
- Muscle weakness, lethargy.
- Arrhythmias.
- Symptoms related to hypocalcemia and hypokalemia, which are resistant to calcium and potassium supplementation, respectively.
- Normal plasma levels range from 1.7–2.4 mg/dL; severe symptoms do not usually occur until levels drop below 1.0 mg/dL.

Hypomagnesemia

Hypomagnesemia is a common abnormality in the ICU (Martin, 2009; Tong, 2005). Total-body magnesium depletion is commonly seen in:

A. Excess loss:
   1. Long-standing diuretics (loop diuretics).
   2. Chronic diabetics, chronic polyuria.
   3. Severe diarrhea or prolonged vomiting, large nasogastric aspirates.
B. Inadequate intake:
   1. Chronic alcoholics or otherwise chronically malnourished (i.e., anorexia, malabsorption).

The development of hypomagnesemia during the course of critical illness is correlated with increased mortality (in patients who were normo- or hypermagnesemic at admission to ICU). There appears to be a poor correlation between ionized and total magnesium levels; however, obtaining an ionized magnesium level has not demonstrated to be a proven beneficial.

Clinical signs and symptoms of hypomagnesemia may be characterized into neuromuscular, cardiovascular, and metabolic (Table 21.1). The hypokalemia seen with hypomagnesemia seems to be related to tubular handling of filtered potassium load. The hypocalcemia is due to inadequate PTH secretion as well as skeletal and gastrointestinal resistance to PTH and Vitamin D.

In the critical-care setting, replacement of magnesium typically occurs via the parenteral route. One gram of magnesium sulfate contains approximately 8 meq of elemental magnesium. It is possible to safely administration of 48 meq of magnesium (approximately 6 gm of magnesium sulfate) over a 24-hour period. Normalization and slight elevation of serum magnesium levels are typically accomplished with this regimen. Redistribution of magnesium is slow, so severely depleted patients may require several replacement attempts before total-body magnesium is replete. Daily magnesium levels should be closely monitored. Renal insufficiency elevates the risk of developing hypermagnesemia. In patients with any degree of renal insufficiency, the dose should be half that for patients without renal impairment, and magnesium level should be closely monitored to avoid significant overshoot.

Hypermagnesemia

Symptomatic hypermagnesemia rarely occurs, even in severe renal failure, except as a consequence of a large magnesium load (in which it may occur even with intact renal function). However, patients with renal failure may develop severe hypermagesemia when exposed to magnesium-containing antacids or laxatives, even in usual therapeutic dosages. Thus, these agents are contraindicated in patients with severe renal failure. Most cases of hypermagnesemia are mild (<3.6 mg/dL, or 1.5 mmol/L) and asymptomatic. However, three types of symptoms may be seen when the plasma magnesium concentration exceeds 4.8 mg/dL (2 mmol/L): neuromuscular; cardiovascular; and hypocalcemia.

Relationship of plasma magnesium and clinical symptoms

Clinically significant hypermagnesemia is an uncommon problem. It is also one of the few abnormalities that may be induced as part of a therapeutic intervention. Clinical evidence of hypermagnesemia begins to manifest as levels start to rise above 3–4 meq/L (3.7–4.8 mg/dL) (Table 21.1). Intravenous calcium (100–200 mg over 5 to 10 minutes) can counteract the effects of acute hypermagnesemia. Dialysis may be considered in severe life threatening hypermagnesemia (with or without renal impairment) (Baker, 2002).

Therapeutic applications of magnesium

Therapeutic applications of magnesium and specifically elevation to supranormal levels include:

1. Pre-eclampsia to prevent the development of eclampsia (empirically for eclampsia treatment).
2. Severe asthma exacerbations.
3. Acute management of Torsade de pointes.

Plasma [Mg2+]	Deep tendon reflexes	Other symptoms/signs
4.8–7.2 mg/dL (2–3 mmol/L)	Diminished	Nausea, flushing, headache, lethargy, and drowsiness
7.3–12 mg/dL (3–5 mmol/L)	Absent	Somnolence, hypocalcemia, hypotension, bradycardia, and ECG changes
>12 mg/dL (>5 mmol/L)	Absent	Muscle paralysis, respiratory paralysis, complete heart block, and cardiac arrest

Bone health and chronic critical illness

The concept of chronic critically ill is an important one in that a significant proportion of patients will endure a prolonged duration of critical illness with concomitant stressors of immobilization, mechanical ventilation, and other organ system support. We have briefly touched on immobilization as a mechanism for hypercalcemiav; in this condition, PTH levels are supressed. This is a demineralizing process and has been associated with pathological nontraumatic fractures. However, bone health is compromised in other ways with chronic critical illness (CCI). A urinary marker of bone turnover (n-telopeptide) is found to be elevated in this population and is associated with vitamin d-deficiency with concomitant nonsuppressed PTH levels. The increase in inflammatory mediators associated with critical illness appears to be important in mediating this process (Van den Berghe, 2003). This potentially places the CCI patient at future risk for osteoporosis-related fractures. Bisphosphonate supplementation has been found to inhibit hyper-resorption in patients with hypercalcemia associated with immobilization. Vitamin D supplementation would theoretically be helpful as 1,25 dihydroxy vitamin D3 suppresses IL-6 and TNF-α, but studies are lacking to guide dosing and timing of initiation (Nierman, 2000; Van den Berghe, 2003). Early initiation of physical activity will also be important in maintaining bone integrity.

Selected references

Baker SB, Worthley LIG. The Essentials of Calcium, Magnesium and Phosphate Metabolism: Part I. Physiology. *Critical Care and Resuscitation: Journal of the Australasian Academy of Critical Care Medicine.* 2002, Dec; 4(4): 301–306.

Baker SB, Worthley LIG. The Essentials of Calcium, Magnesium and Phosphate Metabolism: Part II. Disorders. *Critical Care and Resuscitation: Journal of the Australasian Academy of Critical Care Medicine.* 2002, Dec; 4(4): 307–315.

Berndt TJ, Schiavi S, Kumar R. "Phosphatonins" and the regulation of phosphorous homeostasis. *Am J Physiol Renal Physiol.* 2005; 289:F1170–F1182.

French C, Bellomo R. A rapid intravenous phosphate replacement protocol for critically ill patients. *Critical Care and Resuscitation.* 2004;6:175–179.

Leehey DJ, Ing TS. Correction of hypercalcemia and hypophosphatemia by hemodialysis using a conventional, calcium-containing dialysis solution enriched with phosphorus. *Am J Kidney Dis.* 1997 Feb;*29*(2):288–290.

Martin KJ, Gonzalez EA, Slatopolsky E. Clinical consequences and management of hypo-magnesaemia. *JASN.* 2009;*20*:2291–2295.

Nierman DM, Mechanick JL. Biochemical response to treatment of bone hyperresorption in chronically critically ill Patients. *Chest.* 2000;*118*:761–766.

Tan HK, BellomoR, M'Pis DA, Ronco C. Phosphatemic control during acute renal failure: intermittent hemodialysis versus continuous hemodiafiltration. *Int J Art Organs.* 2001;*24*(4): 186–191.

Tong GM, Rude RK. Magnesium deficiency in critical illness. *J Intensive Care Med.* 2005; *20*:3–17.

Van den Berghe G, Van Roosbroeck D, Vanhove P, et al. Bone turnover in prolonged crit-ical illness: effect of vitamin D. *J Clin Endocrinol Metab.* Oct 2003;*88*(10):4623–4632.

Vincent JL, Jankowski S. Why should ionized calcium be determined in acutely ill patients? *Acta Anaesthesiol Scand.* 1995;*39*:Suppl (107):281–286.

Ziegler R. Hypercalcemic crisis. *J Am Soc Nephrol.* 2001;*12*:s3–s9.

Zivin JR Et Al. Hypocalcaemia: A pervasive metabolic abnormality in the Critically Ill. *Am J Kid Dis.* 2001;*37*(4):689–698.

Chapter 22

Nutrition in the critically ill patient

Juan Ochoa and Jodie Bryk

Nutritional intervention (NI) is pivotal after trauma to improve organ and immune function, as well as to promote wound healing. However, like all interventions, successful implementation involves careful evaluation of risks, benefits, and side effects.

Although NI has been classically described as a "supportive therapy" in trauma patients, a well-designed NI plays an essential role in patient recovery.

Starvation

Average adults and children are able to consume a balanced diet that provides the essential nutrients for organ function in nonstress circumstances. However, when an individual is unable to consume enough nutrients to meet metabolic needs, starvation occurs. There is a physiologic metabolic response to starvation that allows for normal organ function despite inadequate nutrient intake.

Physiologic adaption to starvation

Normal organ function can be maintained for several weeks to months depending on the degree of starvation through adaptive mechanisms. The following protective mechanisms are set-forth to maintain muscle mass and energy stores:

i.   Decreased basal metabolic rate. Energy stores are protected in the starved individual by decreasing metabolic rate to 25 percent of normal. Clinically, a starved individual will have lower heart rates and temperature compared to a fed individual.

ii. Lipid metabolism. An average individual under nonstress circumstances has enough lipid stores to maintain energy needs for several months. During starvation, lipid stores are mobilized and become the principal source of energy.

iii. Glucose metabolism. An average 70-kg individual will require 120 g/day of glucose to maintain central nervous system function. During starvation, glycogen stores are depleted after 24 hours. Protein catabolism is then required to maintain baseline glucose levels.

iv. Decrease nitrogen loss. A normally fed individual loses 15–20 g/d^2 of nitrogen per day, equal to the amount of nitrogen consumed. Starved individuals will initially lose more nitrogen than consumed and utilize endogenous proteins in the liver and muscles to maintain nitrogen balance. However, the rate of nitrogen consumption will decrease by two-thirds during starvation to match the rate of nitrogen consumption and decrease protein depletion.

v. Protein-sparing effect of glucose. Endogenous protein destruction that occurs during starvation produces the gluconeogenic amino acids (such as alanine) required for production of glucose. Small amounts of glucose (roughly 100 g, or 400 calories) will decrease nitrogen losses by 95 percent.

Trauma

a. Adaptation to trauma. The adaptive response to starvation is modified in trauma. Trauma patients have increased catabolism in proportion to the amount of injury sustained. Metabolic alterations in response to trauma include:

i. Increased basal metabolic rate. Basal metabolic rate after trauma increases in proportion to the severity of trauma.

ii. Lipid mobilization. Lipids are the main energy source after trauma. Increased catecholamines after trauma activate triglyceride lipases and promote lipid metabolism.

iii. Hyperglycemia and insulin resistance. Hyperglycemia typically results following trauma and is attributable to excess hepatic gluconeogenesis and decreased glucose storage. Furthermore, insulin release is suppressed in the first few hours after trauma. It is restored in the later phases of trauma recovery; however, hyperglycemia persists secondary to increased insulin resistance.

Hyperglycemia is an independent predictor of poor prognosis. Severe hyperglycemia is associated with decreased neutrophil chemotaxis, phagocytosis, oxidative bursts, and superoxide production. Posttrauma hyperglycemia is worsened by the provision of excessive glucose in dietary formulas.

iv. Increased protein breakdown. Loss of up to 15 percent of lean body mass can occur in the first 10 days after trauma. Increased protein losses occur from wounds, blood, and increased protein catabolism. Protein depletion is a life-threatening condition in severe trauma, and the catabolic rate is resistant to caloric supplementation.

Assessment of malnutrition

In both starvation and trauma, without restoration of nutrition, adaptive responses are eventually exhausted and individuals become malnourished. Severe protein malnutrition is defined as greater than 25–30 percent loss of lean body mass. Malnourished individuals exhibit deterioration of multiple organ functions (including respiratory muscle function), impaired immune response such as T-cell function, and poor wound healing. In stressful circumstances (such as trauma), malnutrition significantly increases morbidity and mortality. Table 22.1 summarizes the four stages of malnutrition.

a. Assessment of malnutrition. Diagnosis of malnutrition is made through multiple means of assessment, including clinical nutrition history, anthropometric measures (such as fat-to-muscle ratios), functional parameters, and biochemical markers (such as prealbumin, albumin).

Multiple calculated formulas have been developed to estimate caloric requirements. These formulas include the Harris-Benedict and the Ireton-Jones Energy expenditure equations (Tables 22.2, 22.3). However, these formulas are often inaccurate, leading to overfeeding or underfeeding a significant proportion of patients.

The gold standard to estimate caloric needs is indirect calorimetry, which evaluates oxygen consumption and carbon dioxide production using metabolic carts.

To determine protein requirements, urine urea nitrogen excretion can be measured to assess protein needs to maintain nitrogen balance.

Table 22.1 The four stages of malnutrition

Well nourished

No physical signs of muscle wasting

No or minimal subcutaneous fat loss

Dietary intake adequate or marginally inadequate for <2 weeks

Mild malnutrition

Mild muscle wasting

Mild subcutaneous fat loss

Inadequate dietary intake of 2–3 weeks

Functional capacity: working suboptimally

Moderate malnutrition

Moderate muscle wasting

Significant subcutaneous fat loss

Inadequate dietary intake 3–5 weeks

Functional capacity: semi-ambulatory, requiring assistance with activities of daily living

Severe malnutrition

Severe muscle wasting

Severe subcutaneous fat loss

Inadequate dietary intake >5 weeks

Functional capacity: minimally ambulatory, bed-ridden

From Pikul J. Degree of preoperative malnutrition is predictive of preoperative morbidity and mortality in liver transplant recipients. *Transplantation*. 1994;57(3):469.

Table 22.2 Harris-Benedict equation

EEE calculation for men	EEE = 66 + (13.7 × weight in kg) + (5 × height in cm)− (6.76 × age in years)
EEE calculation for women	EEE = 655 + (4.35 × weight in pounds) + (4.7 × height in inches) − (4.7 × age in years)
Where EEE is estimated energy expenditure	

Table 22.3 Ireton-Jones equation

EEE = 1925−10 (age in y) + 5(wt in kg) + 281(sex) + 292(trauma) +851(burn)
Where EEE is estimated energy expenditure, sex is 0 for females and 1 for males, trauma is 1 for yes and 0 for no, and burn is 1 for yes and 0 for no

Nutritional interventions

Six categories of nutritional interventions exist; oral intake at will, enteral nutrition, controlled starvation, parenteral nutrition, oral nutrition supplements, and immunonutrition. The option to choose one or more of these forms of nutrition should be carefully evaluated by the physician.

a. Oral intake at will: It is highly psychologically beneficial for the patient to be in charge of their own dietary intake. However, spontaneous dietary intake is frequently interrupted in the hospital for testing and procedures. In addition, the palatability of many in-hospital food preparations is often poor. As a result, patients may progress toward malnutrition. Appropriate monitoring of caloric and protein intake is essential.

b. Enteral nutrition (EN): Enteral nutrition is nutrition provided via feeding tube. Early EN is the gold standard of nutrition interventions and is associated with decreased infection rates, increased wound healing, and decreased hospital length of stay. However, early EN is limited in the presence of shock and poor gut perfusion. Complications may also arise from enteral nutrition. Feeding tube placement, gastrostomies, and jejunostomies are all not without risk. In a recent report, 2 percent of nasoenteral feeding tubes were misplaced within the trachea. Aspiration events are also common and occur more frequently when the tip of the nasoenteric tube is not advanced into the duodenum or jejunum. Bowel necrosis can also occur if aggressive volumes of EN are delivered, especially in the presence of poor bowel perfusion and shock.

c. Controlled starvation: Careful consideration must be given when a patient is made "nothing per oral" (NPO) during hospitalization. Virtually any member of the health-care team is permitted to limit a patient's oral intake despite evidence that proves this is frequently not indicated.

Fasting for 8 hours preoperatively is the norm, although it has been shown that clear liquids up to 2 hours prior to surgery is not associated with adverse affects. After surgery, patients are frequently kept NPO for concerns of postoperative ileus. However, meta-analyses have shown that patients undergoing elective surgery who received early postoperative oral or enteral intake exhibited significantly decreased infection rate, decreased mortality, and decreased anastomotic breakdown. Most patients are able to tolerate oral or enteral intake 24 hours following surgery or trauma.

d. Total parenteral nutrition (TPN): Since 1968, TPN has been a means to provide complete nutritional support in the absence of a functional gastrointestinal tract. Level I evidence of the benefit of TPN exists for the following indications:

   i. Severely malnourished patients who will be undergoing elective surgery.

   ii. Short gut syndrome.

   However, inadequate use of TPN is associated with significantly increased morbidity and mortality. TPN is not indicated when the gastrointestinal tract is intact or during short periods of starvation. In these circumstances, TPN has been shown to increase morbidity and mortality when compared to starvation alone.

e. Oral nutrition supplements: These supplements contain a source of calories and protein in the form of easily absorbed carbohydrates and long-chain fatty acids. There is no evidence to support their use after trauma. In fact, these may be associated with significant complications, including hyperglycemia, and may detract the patient from a regular oral intake.

f. Immunonutrition: Preoperative nutritional supplements containing high concentrations of arginine, glutamine, and omega-3 fatty acids have been classified as immune-enhancing diets. There is Level I evidence that this form of nutrition is associated with better organ perfusion, decreased infection rates, increased tolerance to surgical shock, enhanced T-cell function, and improved nitrogen balance. Currently, preoperative immune-enhancing diets can be advocated for high-risk surgery (such as cardiac surgery, colon resection, or pancreatic resection). Studies have also shown that postoperatively immune-enhancing diets could be of benefit. The data with regards to the benefit of immune-enhancing diets post-trauma is lacking.

Nutrient requirements

a. Caloric requirements: It is traditionally believed that typical metabolic needs of the trauma patient can be met by providing above-baseline requirements (baseline is 25 kcal/kg per day). However, there is no clinical evidence that hypercaloric supplementation improves trauma patient outcomes. In fact, some investigators have recommended feeding below baseline requirements (10–15 kcal/kg per day), a practice known as permissive underfeeding. There is increased morbidity when patient receive excessive calories. Overfeeding increases length of stay on the ventilator and is associated with increased incidence of sepsis. As previously mentioned, the Harris-Benedict and Ireton-Jones have been formulated to determine caloric requirements. A stress factor is added to these formulas in circumstances of trauma or postsurgery to account for the increased basal energy expenditure. Overfeeding results in up to one-third of patients whose caloric requirements are calculated using these formulas. The Canadian Critical Care Nutrition Guidelines have suggested patients should receive approximately 50 percent of traditional caloric goals. The new trend in permissive underfeeding has been associated with decreased length of hospital stay, decreased antibiotic use, and decreased mechanical ventilator days.

b. Carbohydrate requirements: There are several available forms of carbohydrates. They are classified based on complexity (the size of the individual carbohydrate polymers), which determines the need for digestion prior to absorption. Complexity is measured in dextrose equivalents (DE). The DE of readily absorbed dextrose is 100, whereas the DE of cornstarch is 1, which is less readily absorbed. Intermediate values are given to maltodextrin, corn syrup, and modified cornstarch.

c. Protein requirements: Protein provision is essential to minimize loss of lean body mass. Protein synthesis is restored with protein supplementation of 1.5 to 2 g/kg per day, which is 20–30 percent of total caloric nutrient intake. The types of protein commercially available include casein, soy, and whey protein. Predigested protein in the form of simple peptides and individual amino acids are also available and may be beneficial when either digestion or absorption is impaired. No data exists showing one type of protein of particularly greater benefit than the others.

d. Lipid requirements: Lipids provide an essential substrate for cell membrane formation and prostaglandin production. They are the most concentrated energy source of all macronutrients. A diet free of lipids will result in fatty acid deficiency within a few weeks. Thus, the minimum amount of fats provided in the diet should be approximately 2–4 percent of caloric goals. Traditionally, 30 percent of calories delivered to the patient come from lipids; however, this value varies from 15–70 percent in commercially available dietary formulas.

Furthermore, the amount and type of lipid provided in a diet may play distinct physiologic roles in affecting specific organ function.

i. Short-chain fatty acids are produced from broken-down digestible fibers. They may provide a main energy source for the colonic mucosa.

ii. Medium-chain fatty acids are absorbed directly into the blood stream and can be used as energy stores in the absence of carnitine, essential for transport of long-chain fatty acids into mitochondria. Carnitine becomes deficient during critical illness.

iii. Long-chain fatty acids (omega-6 fatty acids) are the traditional source of lipids provided in many diets for critically ill patients and the exclusive source of lipids in intravenous lipid preparations. They are typically found in corn oil.

iv. Omega-3 fatty acids through inhibition of prostaglandin E2 in favor of prostaglandin E3 are said to be anti-inflammatory. These acids are contained in fish oil and frequently provided to patients with acute respiratory distress syndrome.

e. Micronutrients: Little is known of dietary supplementation of micronutrients (vitamins and minerals) in trauma and critical illness. In most cases, micronutrients are provided in quantities sufficient to meet recommended dietary allowance (RDA). It is known that dietary levels of vitamin C significantly decrease after trauma and hemorrhagic shock. Preliminary trials suggest that the administration of supraphysiologic quantities of vitamin C as part of resuscitation protocol may have significantly improve outcomes. Supplemental zinc and selenium are also frequently given to patients with large wounds and decubitus ulcers.

Nutrition in special patient populations

a. Burn patients: Burn patients exhibit higher metabolic rates and require caloric provision primarily in the form of carbohydrates. Most severe burn patient are cared for in burn units in which specialized nutritional support is available.

b. Obese patients: Obese patients may exhibit occult but significant nutritional deficiencies. Accumulating evidence suggests that obese patients may benefit from the use of hypocaloric high protein diets.

c. Elderly patients: Elderly patients have increased metabolic problems providing for significant challenge in nutritional intervention. Many are typically malnourished at baseline, and trauma and surgery exacerbate this. Hyperglycemia is frequent.

Clinical guidelines

The Eastern Association of the Surgery of Trauma (EAST) has created guidelines to assist clinician in the formulations of NI in trauma. Other associations have created guidelines to assist in the formulation of NI, and these guidelines serve to provide practical suggestions toward the approach of NI. Practical suggestions are presented next:

a. Does the patient require nutritional intervention? If short periods of starvation are tolerated in a previously healthy patient, then NI it not warranted. However, NI is indicated in patients who cannot eat by themselves. If the period of starvation is anticipated to last longer than 7 days, then NI should be considered.

b. Enteral nutrition is strongly favored over TPN. Starting TPN when EN is not meeting caloric goal is discouraged. Again, TPN is only indicated in those with severe malnutrition who are to undergo elective surgery or those with a nonfunctional gastrointestinal tract. Furthermore, surgical manipulation of the gastrointestinal tract is not a contraindication to enteral nutrition.

c. Enteral nutrition should be started within 24 hours of surgery or trauma. Achievement of caloric goals early is unimportant; however, to maintain gastrointestinal functions, a small rate of EN (trickle feed) should be attempted. However, EN is contraindicated when the patient is in shock, and when there is associated bowel necrosis and bowel ischemia.

d. Do not overfeed critically ill patients. Overfeeding patient is associated with significant morbidity and possible increased mortality. Consider using a hypocaloric diet, especially when ordering TPN.

e. Monitor nutritional interventions closely. Avoid hyperglycemia and hyperlipidemia in the critically ill patient. A low albumin and prealbumin may not always indicate malnutrition, but rather serve as markers of the severity of disease. Overfeeding the patient with low level of albumin and prealbumin will not hasten the patient's recovery.

f. Most patients can be fed a standard polymeric diet. Specialized nutritional formulas should be used in consultation with a nutritional support team. Immune-enhancing diets can be used carefully and early for short periods of time (5–10 days). However, immune-enhancing diets should be avoided in septic patients.

Suggested readings

Bertolini G, Iapichino G, Radrissani D, et al. Early enteral immunonutrition in the patients with severe sepsis: Results of an interim analysis of a randomized multicentre clinical trial. *Intens Care Med.* 2003;29:671.

Bower RH, Cerra FB, Bershadsky B. Early enteral administration of a formula supplemented with arginine, nucleotides, and fish oil in intensive care unit patients: Results of a multicenter, prospective randomized clinical trial. *Crit Care Med.* 1995;23:436.

Brown R, Hunt H, Mowatt-Larssen C, Kudsk K. Comparison of specialized and standard enteral formulas in trauma patients. *Pharmacotherapy.* 1994;14:314.

Cresci GA. Nutrition support in trauma. In: Gottschlich MM, ed. *The Science and Practice of Nutrition Support: A Case-Based Core Curriculum.* Dubuque, Iowa: Kendall/Hunt Publishing Co; 2001:445.

Dickerson RN, Boschert KJ, Kudsk KA, et al. Hypocaloric enteral tube feeding in critically ill obese patients. *Nutrition.* 2002;*18*:241.

Dickerson RN, Rosato EF, Mullen JL. Net protein anabolism with hypocaloric parenteral nutrition in obese stresses patients. *Am J Clin Nutr.* 1986;*44*:747.

Frankenfield DC. Correlation between measured energy expenditure and clinically obtain variables in trauma and sepsis. *J Trauma.* 1994;*18*:398.

Frankenfield DC. Energy and macrosubstrate requirements. In: Gottschlich MM, ed. *The Science and Practice of Nutrition Support: A Case-Based Core Curriculum.* Dubuque, Iowa: Kendall/Hunt Publishing Co; 2001:31.

Freund E, Freund O. Beitrage zum Stoffwechsel im Hungerzustand. *Med Klin.* 1901;*15*:69.

Fuhrman PM. Hepatic proteins and nutrition assessment. *Jam Diet Assoc.* 2004;*104*:1258.

Hasselgren PO, Fisher JE. Counter-regulatory hormones and mechanisms in amino acid metabolism with special reference to the catabolic response in skeletal muscle. *Curr Opin Nutr Metab Care.* 1999;*2*(1):9.

Hoffer LJ. Starvation. In: Shils ME, Olson JA, Shike M, eds. *Modern Nutrition in Health and Disease.* Philadelphia. Pa: Lea & Febinger; 1994:927.

Ireton-Jones CS. Equation for estimating energy expenditure in burn patients with special reference e to ventilator status. *J Burn Care Rehab.* 1992;*13*(3):330–333.

Keys A. Basal metabolism. In: *The Biology of Human Starvation.* St. Paul, Minn: North Central Publishing Co; 1950:303.

Krishnan JA, Parce PB, Martinez A, et al. Caloric intake in medical ICU patients: Consistency of care with guideline and relationship to clinical outcomes. *Chest.* 2003; *124*:297.

Kudsk KA, Minard G, Croce MA, et al. A randomized trial of isonitrogenous enteral diets after severe trauma: An immune-enhancing diet reduces septic complications. *Ann Surg.* 1996;*224*:531.

Lewis SJ, Egger M, Sylvester PA, et al. Early enteral feeding versus "nil by mouth" after gastrointestinal surgery: Systemic review and meta-analysis of controlled trials. *BMJ.* 2001;*323*:773.

Lin E, Calvano SE, Lowry SF. Systemic response to injury and metabolic support. In: Brunicardi FC, Andersen DK, Billiar TR, et al. *Schwartz's Principles of Surgery.* New York: McGraw-Hill Medical Publishing Div; 2005:3.

Long CL. Metabolic response to injury and illness: Estimation of energy and protein needs from indirect calorimetry and nitrogen balance. *J Parenter Enteral Nutr.* 1979;*3*:452.

Long CL. Effect of amino acid infusion on glucose production in trauma patient. *J Trauma.* 1996;*40*:335.

Marderstein EL, Simmons RL, Ochoa JB. Patient Safety: Effect of institutional protocols on adverse events related to feeding tube placement in the critically ill. *J Am Coll Surg.* 2004;*199*:39.

Marik PE, Pinsky M. Death by parenteral nutrition. *Intens Case Med.* 2003;*29*:867.

McClave SA, Snider HL. Use of indirect calorimetry in clinical nutrition. *Nutr Clin Pract.* 1992;*7*(5):207–221.

Moore FA, Moore EE, Kudsk KA. Clinical benefits of immune enhancing diet for early postinjury enteral feeding. *J Trauma.* 1994;*37*:607.

Piccione VA, LeVeen HH. Prehepatic hyperalimentation. *Surgery.* 1987;*87*:263.

Pikul J. Degree of preoperative malnutrition is predictive of preoperative morbidity and mortality in liver transplant recipients. *Transplantation*. 1994;*57*(3):469.

Sandstrom R, Drott C, Hyltander A, et al. The effect of postoperative intravenous feeding (TPN) on outcome following major surgery evaluated in a randomized study. *Ann Surg*. 1993;*217*:185.

Tepaske R, Velthuis H. Effect of preoperative oral immune-enhancing nutritional supplement on patient at high risk of infection after cardiac surgery: A randomized placebo-controlled trial. *Lancet*. 2001;*358*:696.

Zaloga GP. Permissive underfeeding. *New Horiz*. 1994;*2*:257.

Index

A

Abdominal compartment
    syndrome
    acute kidney injury in, 6
    management of, 8
Abortion
    hemorrhage in, 115t
    septic, 114
Abruptio placenta, 115t
Absorption, drug, 57–58
Acebutolol, 65t
ACE inhibitors
    with chronic kidney disease,
        32, 34
    for critically ill with kidney
        disease, 66
    decreased kidney function
        on, 62t
Acid-base disorders, 131–136
    diagnosis of, 131, 132t
    management of, 132
    metabolic, 132–135, 132t
    pathogenesis of, 131
    respiratory, 132t, 135–136
Acidosis
    in diabetic, 165
    lactic, 132–134, 132t
    from metformin, 165–166
    renal replacement therapy
        for, 72, 134
    metabolic, 132–134, 132t
    renal replacement therapy
        for, 72
    respiratory, 132t, 135–136
ACTH-secreting pituitary
    adenomas, 180
Acute adrenal crisis, 178, 180
Acute fatty liver of pregnancy
    (AFLP), 112–113, 113t
Acute glomerulonephritis,
    in acute kidney injury,
    17–18, 18t
Acute kidney injury (AKI),
    3–10. See also specific topics
    acute glomerulonephritis in,
        17–18, 18t
    vs. acute renal failure, 3
    acute tubulointerstitial
        nephritis in, 16–17, 123
    after cardiac surgery, 6,
        11–13 (See also Cardiac
        surgery)
    chronic kidney disease and,
        in ICU, 30

classification of, 3–4, 4f,
    100–101
clinical consequences of, 9,
    9t–10t
definition of, 3, 100, 100t,
    102
etiology of, 5–7
    with cirrhosis, 103
    Goodpasture syndrome in,
        20–22
    hemolytic-uremic syndrome
        in, 18–20
    hypotension in, 5–6
    in ICU, 30
    incidence and progression
        of, 4
    with liver disease, 100–101,
        100t
management of, 7–8
    for abdominal
        compartment syndrome,
        8
    for glomerular disease, 7
    hemodynamic, 7
    for interstitial nephritis, 8
    renal replacement therapy
        in, 8–9
    for urinary tract
        obstruction, 7
    oliguria in, 3
    pharmacologic therapy for
        shock in, 49–55
        diuretics in, 53–55
        mannitol in, 53
        N-acetyl-cysteine in, 53
        vasodilators and atrial
            natriuretic peptide in,
            52–53
        vasopressors and inotropes
            in, 50–52, 50t–51t
        volume expansion in, 49–50
    postoperative, 6
    on pulmonary function,
        92–93, 92f
    from radiocontrast agents,
        6, 7t, 13–16 (See also
        Radiocontrast agents,
        AKI from)
    renal replacement therapy
        in, 77–90 (See also Renal
        replacement therapy
        (RRT), in AKI)
    risk factors for, 5
    sepsis in, 5, 23–27 (See also
        Sepsis)

volume-responsive, 5
Acute lung injury (ALI), 91
Acute renal failure (ARF)
    vs. acute kidney injury, 3
    management of, 7–8 (See
        also Acute kidney injury
        (AKI), management of)
Acute respiratory distress
    syndrome (ARDS), 91
Acute tubulointerstitial
    nephritis (ATIN)
    in AKI, 16–17
    in children, 123
Acyclovir
    for critically ill with kidney
        disease, 60t–61t, 65
    decreased kidney function
        on, 60t
Addison's disease, 177–179
Adenoma
    ACTH-secreting pituitary,
        180
    adrenal, 181
Adrenal adenoma, 181
Adrenal cortex, 177
Adrenal crisis, acute, 178, 180
Adrenal disease, 177–183
    androgen-secreting tumors
        and congenital adrenal
        hyperplasia, 182–183
    hypercortisolism (Cushing's
        syndrome), 180–181
    hypothalamic-pituitary-
        adrenal axis in, 177,
        178f
    prevalence of, 177
    primary adrenal insufficiency
        (Addison's disease),
        177–179
    primary aldosteronism
        (Conn syndrome),
        180–181
    secondary adrenal
        insufficiency, 179–180
Adrenal glands, 177
Adrenal insufficiency
    primary, 177–179
    relative, 178–180
    secondary, 179–180
Adrenal medulla, 177
Advance care planning, 36
Alarms, machine, on fluid
    management, 42
Albumin with diuretics, in AKI,
    54–55

Aldosteronism, primary, 181–182
Alemtuzumab, 154t
Alkalosis
    metabolic, 132t, 134–135
    respiratory, 132t, 135–136
Allopurinol, 65t
Alpha-adrenergic stimulation, 50t
Aminoglycosides
    with chronic kidney disease, 33
    for critically ill with kidney disease, 60t–61t, 65
    decreased kidney function on, 61t
Amniotic fluid embolus, 116
Analgesics, 64
Anaphylactoid syndrome of pregnancy, 116
Androgen-secreting tumors, 182–183
Anemia management, with chronic kidney disease, 35
Angiotensin receptor blockers (ARBs), 32, 34
Antibody preparations, 154t–155t
Anticoagulants
    for critically ill with kidney disease, 64
    decreased kidney function on, 60t
Anti-glomerular basement membrane disease, AKI in, 20–22
Antimetabolites, 153t
Antimicrobials
    for critically ill with kidney disease, 64–65
    decreased kidney function on, 60t–61t
Antithymocyte globulins, 154t
Antivirals, 60t–61t, 65
Apoptosis, 93
Arginine vasopressin (AVP)
    for AKI prevention in shock, 51
    for AKI with cirrhosis, 103t, 104
    for septic shock, 25–26
Arterio-venous blood circuits, 79
Atenolol
    for critically ill with kidney disease, 66
    decreased kidney function on, 62t
Atgam, 154t
Atrial natriuretic peptide (ANP), for shock, 52–53
Azathioprine, 153t
Azotemia, 71

B

Bacterial infections, after renal transplantation, 148–149, 149f
Basliximab, 155t
Benzodiazepines, 62t
Beta-adrenergic stimulation, 50t
Beta-blockers
    for critically ill with kidney disease, 66
    decreased kidney function on, 62t
Beta-lactam antibiotics, 60t–61t, 64
Bicarbonate, for diabetic ketoacidosis, 163t, 165
Bivalirudin
    for critically ill with kidney disease, 64
    decreased kidney function on, 60t
Bleeding, after renal transplantation, 148
Blood pressure measurements, in children, 128
Bone health, in chronic critical illness, 198
Bortezomib, 155t
Bumetanide dosing, 71t
Burn patients, nutrition in, 207

C

Calcineurin inhibitors (CNIs), 152t
Calcium
    concentration of, 185
    role of, 185
Calcium disorders
    in critically ill, 185–186, 192–194
    differential diagnosis of, 186, 190t
    hypercalcemia, 187t–188t, 192–194, 193t
    hypocalcemia, 186, 187t, 190t, 192
    after renal transplant, 146–148, 147t
    hypercalcemia, 192–194
    causes of, 192
    clinical manifestations of, 187t–188t, 192
    definition of, 192
    differential diagnosis of, 190t
    from immobilization, 198
    management of, 187t–188t, 192–194, 193t
    after renal transplant, 146–148, 147t
    symptoms of, 192
    hypocalcemia, 186, 192
    causes of, 186
    clinical manifestations of, 187t
    differential diagnosis of, 186, 187t, 190t
    management of, 187t, 192
    prevalence of, ICU, 186
    after renal transplant, 146–148, 147t
Caloric requirements, 205–206
Carbepenems, 61t
Carbohydrate requirements, 206
Cardiac surgery
    acute kidney injury after, 6, 11–13
    diagnosis and biomarkers for, 12
    epidemiology of, 11
    pathogenesis of, 11–12
    risk factors and prevention of, 12–13, 12t
    chronic kidney disease after, 31
Cardiac troponins, 32
Cardiovascular agents. See also specific agents
    for critically ill with kidney disease, 66
    decreased kidney function on, 62t
Cardiovascular disease. See also specific types
    after renal transplant, 145, 145t
Cardiovascular insufficiency, 43–44
Catecholamines, for septic shock, 25–26
CdDPTA clearance, 98t
Cephalosporins, decreased kidney function on, 61t
Children. See Pediatrics, renal disorders in
Chlorothiazide
    dosing of, 71t
    for volume overload, 70–71
Chorioamnionitis, 114
Chronic critical illness, bone health and, 198
Chronic kidney disease (CKD). See also specific topics
    acute kidney injury and, in ICU, 30
    classification of, 30t
    in critically ill, 29–36 (See also Critically illness, chronic kidney disease in)

definition of, 29
epidemiology of, 29
patient outcomes with, 30
renal outcomes with, 30
Chvostek's sign, 186
Cirrhosis, with acute kidney
  injury, 99–105
  acute kidney injury in,
    100–101, 100t
  approach to patient in,
    102–103
  hepatorenal syndrome in,
    101–102, 102t
  management of, 103–105,
    103t, 105t (See also
    Combined kidney-liver
    failure)
  renal function assessment in,
    97–100, 98t
  ancillary testing in, 99–100
  creatine based equations
    in, 99
  glomerular filtration rate
    in, 97, 98t
  serum creatine in, 98t, 99
Citrate toxicity, hypocalcemia
  with, 186, 192
Clearance, liver, 98t
Coarctation of the aorta,
  128–129
Cockcroft Gault equation,
  99
Codeine, 64, 65t
Combined kidney-liver failure,
  99–105
  acute kidney injury in liver
    disease patients in,
    100–101, 100t
  approach to patient with,
    102–103
  hepatorenal syndrome in,
    101–102, 102t
  management of, 103–105
  extracorporeal therapy in,
    104–105
  liver transplantation in,
    105, 105t
  pharmacologic, 103–104,
    103t
  renal replacement therapy
    in, 105
  transjugular intrahepatic
    portosystemic shunt
    in, 104
  renal function assessment in,
    97–100, 98t
  ancillary testing in, 99–100
  creatine based equations
    in, 99
  glomerular filtration rate
    in, 97, 98t
  serum creatine in, 98t, 99

Combined kidney-lung failure,
  91–94
  acute kidney failure on
    pulmonary function in,
    92, 92f
  acute lung injury in
    definition and classification
      of, 91
    on renal function, 92–94,
      94f
    pathophysiology of, 92–93,
      92f
    on survival, 91
Compartment syndrome,
  abdominal
  acute kidney injury in, 6
  management of, 8
Congenital adrenal
  hyperplasia, 182–183
Congenital disorders of the
  kidney, 123–125
  hydronephrosis, 123
  multicystic dysplastic kidney,
    124–125
  nephronophthisis, 125
  posterior urethral valves,
    124
  prune belly syndrome, 124
  ureteropelvic junction
    obstruction, 124
Congenital nephrotic
  syndrome (CNS), 126–127
Congenital nephrotic
  syndrome of Finnish type,
  126
Congestive heart failure,
  chronic kidney disease
  with, 31
Conn syndrome, 181–182
Continuous renal replacement
  therapy (CRRT)
  for AKI with cirrhosis, 105
  fluid balance in, 39, 40,
    40t, 41t (See also Fluid
    management)
  fluid management in,
    39–42 (See also Fluid
    management)
  hemodynamic stability in, 85
  with hypercalcemia, 193
  off-time in, 41–42
  for severe sepsis and septic
    shock, 89
Contrast-induced
  nephropathy, 6, 7t, 13–16.
  See also Radiocontrast
  agents, AKI from
  chronic kidney disease from,
    31–32
  renal replacement therapy
    for, 72–73, 74t
Contrast nephropathy, 73

Controlled starvation,
  204–205
Convection, 82
Convective treatments, 81–82
Corticosteroids, for septic
  shock, 26
COX-2 inhibitors, 33
Creatine assessment, serum,
  98t, 99
CrEDTA clearance, 98t
Critical illness. See also specific
  disorders
  bone health and, 198
  diabetes mellitus on
    diabetes in, 159–160
    hyperglycemia and glucose
      control in, 160–161
  nutrition in, 201–208
    (See also Nutrition, in
    critically ill)
Critically illness, chronic
  kidney disease in, 29–36
  after cardiac surgery, 31
  classification of, 30, 30t
  with congestive heart
    failure, 31
  with contrast-induced
    nephropathy, 31–32
  epidemiology of, 30
  management of
    advance care planning in, 36
    for anemia, 35
    deep vein thrombosis
      prophylaxis in, 35
    glucose control in, 36
    protein intake in, 36
    resuscitation in, initial, 35
    stress ulcer prophylaxis in, 35
  outcomes in, 30
  sedation and neuromuscular
    blockade in, 36
  special considerations in
    ACE inhibitors and
      angiotensin receptor
      blockers in, 32, 34
    cardiac troponins in, 32
    diuretics in, 33–34
    hydroxyethyl starch in,
      34–35
    intravenous immune
      globulin in, 34
    nephrotoxins in, 32–33
Crystal nephropathy, 6
Cushing's syndrome, 180–181
Cyclophosphamide, 153t
Cyclosporine, 152t
Cystatin C, serum, 98t
Cytokines
  in AKI and acute lung
    injury, 92
  renal replacement therapy
    for, 74

D

Dabigatran, 64
Daclizumab, 155t
Dalteparin
  for critically ill with kidney disease, 64
  decreased kidney function on, 60t
Deep vein thrombosis (DVT) prophylaxis, 35
Delayed graft function (DGF), renal, 143, 144t
Demineralization, from immobilization, 198
Denys-Drash syndrome, 127
Desirudin
  for critically ill with kidney disease, 64
  decreased kidney function on, 60t
Dexmedetomidine, 66
Dextrose equivalents (DE), 206
D+ HUS, 119–120
D- HUS, 120–121
Diabetes mellitus, 159–166
  on critical illness diabetes in, 159–160
  hyperglycemia and glucose control in, 160–161
  epidemiology of, 159
  hyperglycemic crisis and diabetic ketoacidosis or HHC in, 161–165
    (See also Diabetic ketoacidosis (DKA); Hyperglycemic hyperosmolar coma (HHC))
  metformin and lactic acidosis in, 165–166
Diabetic ketoacidosis (DKA), 161–165
  diagnosis of, 161–162, 162t
  management of
    criteria for resolution of, 164t, 165
    electrolyte correction in, 163t, 165
    fluid therapy in, 163t, 164
    insulin in, 163t, 164–165
    principles of, 163–164, 163t
  pathogenesis of, 161
  precipitating event in, 163
  symptoms and laboratory findings in, 162
Dialysis. See also specific types
  with hypercalcemia, 193
  in pregnancy, 111
Dialyzers, 81
Diazepam, 62t

Diffusion, in renal replacement therapies, 82
Digoxin
  with chronic kidney disease, 32
  for critically ill with kidney disease, 66
  decreased kidney function on, 62t
Distribution, drug, 58
Diuretics. See also specific types
  in acute kidney injury
    adverse effects of, 55
    co-administration of albumin with, 54–55
    pharmacology of, 54
    resistance in, 55
  for acute kidney injury prevention in shock, 53–55
    uses of, 53–54
  with chronic kidney disease, 33–34
  for critically ill with kidney disease, 66
  decreased kidney function on, 63t
  dosing of, 71t
  for volume overload, 70–71
Dobutamine, for shock, for AKI prevention, 51t
Dopamine
  for septic shock, 25
  for shock, for AKI prevention, 51, 51t
Dopaminergic stimulation, 50t
Drug dosing, in kidney disease, 57–68
  adjustment strategies in, 66–68
  drug selection in, 64–66
    of analgesics, 64
    of anticoagulants, 64
    of antimicrobials, 64–65
    of cardiovascular agents, 66
    of diuretics, 66
    other considerations in, 66
    of sedatives, 66
  pharmacokinetics of, 57–63
    absorption in, 57–58
    distribution in, 58
    excretion in, 59, 63
    metabolism in, 58
    for selected drugs, 60t–63t
Drug-drug interactions, with renal transplant medications, 150t–151t
Drug removal, renal replacement therapy for, 72, 73t

Drug selection, in kidney disease, 64–66
  of analgesics, 64
  of anticoagulants, 64
  of antimicrobials, 64–65
  of cardiovascular agents, 66
  of diuretics, 66
  other considerations in, 66
  of sedatives, 66
Dry weight, 40
Dysnatremias, 137–141
  hypernatremia, 137–138, 138t
  hyponatremia, 138–141

E

Early Goal Directed Therapy (EGDT) study, 24, 24f
Ectopic pregnancy, hemorrhage in, 115t
Edema, 40
Effluent, 39
Elderly, nutrition in, 207
Electrolyte disorders, 137–142. See also Calcium disorders; specific types
  in diabetic ketoacidosis and hyperglycemic hyperosmolar coma, 165
  dysnatremias, in, 137–141
    hypernatremia, 137–138, 138t
    hyponatremia, 138–141 (See also Hyponatremia)
  electrolyte losses in, 137t
  potassium
    hyperkalemia, 71–72, 76, 141–142, 146t
    hypokalemia, 141–142, 146–148, 147t, 165
    after renal transplant, 146–148, 146t–147t
Endotoxin
  polymyxin B for, 90
  in sepsis syndrome, 89–90
Enoxaparin, 60t
Enteral nutrition (EN), 204
Epinephrine
  for AKI prevention in shock, 51, 51t
  for septic shock, 25
Ethylene glycol poisoning, 73t
Excretion, drug, 59, 63, 65t
Extracorporeal therapy, for AKI with cirrhosis, 104–105

F

Fatty acids
  long-chain, 207
  medium-chain, 207

omega-3, 207
short-chain, 206
Fenoldopam, for AKI
prevention in shock, 52
Fentanyl, 64
Fibroblast growth factor-23
(FGF-23), 195
Filtration, plasma, with
hemadsorption, 89
Fluconazole
for critically ill with kidney
disease, 60t–61t, 65
decreased kidney function
on, 61t
Fluid balance
in continuous renal
replacement therapy, 39,
40, 40t, 41t
patient, 39
Fluid management, 39–42
benefits of, 42
dry weight in, 40
edema in, 40
effluent in, 39
fluid status assessment
in, 40
importance of, 39
outcomes of, expected, 41
patient fluid balance in, 39
potential problems in, 41–42
practical considerations in,
40–41, 41t
Fluid overload, 39
on mortality, 87, 87f
Fluid-responsive acute kidney
injury, 5
Fluid responsiveness
assessment, during
spontaneous breathing, 46
Fluid status assessment, 40
Fluoroquinolones
for critically ill with kidney
disease, 60t–61t, 65
decreased kidney function
on, 61t
Fondaparinux
for critically ill with kidney
disease, 64
decreased kidney function
on, 60t
Frasier syndrome, 127
Functional hemodynamic
monitoring, 43–47
applicability of, 47
cardiovascular insufficiency
identification in, 43–44
definition of, 43
fluid responsiveness
assessment in, during
spontaneous breathing,
46
vs. monitoring, 43

volume responsiveness in,
44–45, 45t
Fungal infections, after renal
transplantation, 148–149,
149f
Furosemide
dosing of, 71t
for volume overload,
70–71

G

Gadolinium toxicity, 15–16
Ganciclovir
for critically ill with kidney
disease, 60t–61t, 65
decreased kidney function
on, 61t
Glomerular disease, acute
kidney injury from, 6
Glomerular filtration rate
(GFR) assessment, 97, 98t
Glomerulonephritis, acute,
17–18, 18t
Glomerulonephritis, in
children
acute, 121–123
poststreptococcal
glomerulonephritis,
121–122
rapidly progressive
glomerulonephritis,
122–123
membranoproliferative
glomerulonephritis, 122
primary, 122
Glucose control
with chronic kidney disease,
36
in diabetics in critical illness,
160–161
Glycine vasopressin, for AKI
prevention in shock, 51
Goodpasture syndrome, AKI
in, 20–22

H

Harris-Benedict equation, 203,
204t, 206
HELLP syndrome, 111–112,
112t, 113t
Hemadsorption, plasma
filtration with, 89
Hemodialysis, in pregnancy,
111
Hemodynamic monitoring,
functional, 43–47
applicability of, 47
cardiovascular insufficiency
identification in, 43–44
definition of, 43

fluid responsiveness
assessment in, during
spontaneous breathing,
46
vs. monitoring, 43
volume responsiveness in,
44–45, 45t
Hemodynamic stability, 85–88
in continuous renal
replacement therapy, 85
fluid overload and mortality
in, 87, 87f
in intermittent hemodialysis,
85–87
Hemofilters, 81
Hemofiltration
high-volume, 89
of large molecules, 88–90
Hemolytic uremic syndrome
(HUS)
AKI in, 6, 18–20
in children
D- HUS (atypical HUS),
120–121
D+ HUS (typical HUS),
119–120
in pregnancy, 112–113, 113t
Hemorrhage
in pregnancy, 114, 115t
after renal transplantation,
148
Heparin, 64
Hepatorenal syndrome,
101–102, 102t. See also
Combined kidney-liver
failure
High-volume hemofiltration
(HVHF), 89
H2-receptor antagonists
for critically ill with kidney
disease, 66
decreased kidney function
on, 63t
Hydromorphone, 64
Hydronephrosis, 123
Hydroxyethyl, 34–35
Hypercalcemia, 192–194
causes of, 192
clinical manifestations of,
187t–188t, 192
definition of, 192
differential diagnosis of, 190t
from immobilization, 198
management of, 187t–188t,
192–194, 193t
after renal transplant,
146–148, 147t
symptoms of, 192
Hyperchloremia, 133–134
Hypercoagulable state, after
renal transplantation, 148
Hypercortisolism, 180–181

Hyperglycemia, in diabetics with critical illness, 160–161
Hyperglycemic hyperosmolar coma (HHC), 161–165
  diagnosis of, 161–162, 162t
  management of
    criteria for resolution of, 164t, 165
    electrolyte correction in, 163t, 165
    fluid therapy in, 163t, 164
    insulin in, 163t, 164–165
    principles of, 163–164, 163t
  pathogenesis of, 161
  precipitating event in, 163
  symptoms and laboratory findings in, 162
Hyperkalemia, 141
  management of, initial, 71–72
  renal replacement therapy for, 71–72, 76
  after renal transplant, 146–148, 146t
  risks of, 71
  signs of, 71
Hypermagnesemia, 197, 197t
  clinical manifestations of, 189t, 197
  differential diagnosis of, 191t
  management of, 189t, 197–198
Hypernatremia, 137–138, 138t
Hyperparathyroidism, hypercalcemia from, 192
Hyperphosphatemia, 188t–189t, 194–195
  causes of, 194
  clinical manifestations of, 188t–189t, 195
  definition of, 195
  differential diagnosis of, 191t
  hypocalcemia with, 186
  management of, 188t–189t, 195
  after renal transplant, 146–148, 147t
Hypertension
  in children, 127–130
    blood pressure measurements in, 128
    coarctation of the aorta in, 128–129
    hypertensive urgencies and emergencies in, 130
    pheochromocytoma or paraganglioma in, 129
    renal artery stenosis in, 128
    renal parenchymal disease in, 129

  intracranial, renal replacement therapy for, 76
  pulmonary, after renal transplant, 145–146
  after renal transplantation, 149, 150t
Hypertensive disorders of pregnancy, 111–114
  acute fatty liver of pregnancy in, 112–113
  preeclampsia and HELLP syndrome in, 111–112, 112t, 113t
Hypertensive urgencies and emergencies, in children, 130
Hyperthyroidism, preexisting and newly diagnosed, 172
Hypocalcemia, 186, 187t, 192
  causes of, 186
  clinical manifestations of, 187t
  differential diagnosis of, 186, 187t, 190t
  management of, 187t, 192
  prevalence of, ICU, 186
  after renal transplant, 146–148, 147t
Hypokalemia, 141–142
  in diabetic, 165
  after renal transplant, 146–148, 147t
Hypomagnesemia, 196–197
  causes of, 196
  clinical manifestations of, 189t, 196
  differential diagnosis of, 191t
  management of, 189t, 197
  after renal transplant, 146–148, 147t
Hyponatremia, 138–141
  causes of, 140–141, 140t
  extracellular fluid volume depletion in, 139
  extracellular fluid volume excess in, 139
  general points on, 140
  rate and degree of correction of, 139
  signs and symptoms of, 138
  syndrome of inappropriate ADH secretion in, 139–141
Hypophosphatemia, 188t–189t, 194
  clinical manifestations of, 188t, 194
  differential diagnosis of, 191t
  hypocalcemia with, 186
  management of, 188t, 194

  after renal transplant, 146–148, 147t
Hypotension
  acute kidney injury from, 5–6
  reducing risk of, renal replacement therapy for, 75–76
Hypothalamic-pituitary-adrenal axis, 177, 178f
Hypothyroidism
  myxedema coma, 173–174
  preexisting, 171–172

I

Idiopathic nephrotic syndrome (INS), 125–126
Immobilization, hypercalcemia from, 198
Immunonutrition, 205
Incidentaloma, 181
Induced abortion, hemorrhage in, 115t
Infections. See also specific types
  in pregnancy, 114–116
  after renal transplantation, 148–149, 149f
Inotropes, for AKI prevention in shock, 50–52, 50–51t
Insulin
  decreased kidney function on, 63t
  for diabetic ketoacidosis, 163t, 164–165
  for hyperglycemic hyperosmolar coma, 163t, 164–165
Intermittent hemodialysis (IHD), 79t
  hemodynamic stability in, 85–87
Intermittent positive-pressure ventilation (IPPV), left-ventricular output in, 44–45, 45t
Interstitial nephritis, 8
Intracranial hypertension, renal replacement therapy for, 76
Intrapartum hemorrhage, 115t
Intravenous immune (IVIG)
  with chronic kidney disease, 34
  for renal transplantation, 154t
Inulin clearance, 98t
Iothalamate clearance, 98t
Ireton-Jones equation, 203, 204t

Isopropanol poisoning, renal replacement therapy for, 73t
Isoproterenol, 51t
Itraconazole
  for critically ill with kidney disease, 60t–61t, 65
  decreased kidney function on, 61t

K

Ketoacidosis, 133
Ketorolac, 63t
Kidney disease. See specific types
Kidney injury, acute. See Acute kidney injury (AKI)
Kidney-liver failure, combined, 99–105
  approach to patient with, 102–103
  hepatorenal syndrome in, 101–102, 102t
  management of, 103–105, 103t, 105t (See also Combined kidney-liver failure)
  renal function assessment in, 97–100, 98t
    ancillary testing in, 99–100
    creatine based equations in, 99
    glomerular filtration rate in, 97, 98t
    serum creatine in, 98t, 99
Kidney-lung failure, combined, 91–94
  acute kidney failure on pulmonary function in, 92, 92f
  acute lung injury in
    definition and classification of, 91
    on renal function, 92–94, 94f
    pathophysiology of, 92–93, 92f
    on survival, 91
Kidney transplantation, ICU management of. See Renal transplantation

L

Lactic acidosis, 132–134, 132t
  from metformin, 165–166
  renal replacement therapy for, 72, 134
Large-molecule hemofiltration, 88–90
Leflunimide, 153t

Left-ventricular output, in positive-pressure ventilation, 44–45, 45t
Lepirudin
  for critically ill with kidney disease, 64
  decreased kidney function on, 60t
Leukocyte trafficking and recruitment, in combined kidney-lung failure, 93
Levothyroxine, 171
Liothyronine, 171
Lipid requirements, 206–207
Lithium poisoning, renal replacement therapy for, 73t
Liver disease (cirrhosis)
  acute kidney injury with, 100–101, 100t
  renal function assessment in, 97–100, 98t (See also under Cirrhosis)
Liver transplantation, for AKI with cirrhosis, 105, 105t
Long-chain fatty acids, 207
Loop diuretics
  with acute kidney injury
    adverse effects of, 55
    co-administration of albumin with, 54–55
    pharmacology of, 54
    resistance in, 55
  with chronic kidney disease, 33–34
  for critically ill with kidney disease, 66
  decreased kidney function on, 63t
  dosing of, 71t
  for volume overload, 70–71
Lorazepam
  for critically ill with kidney disease, 66
  decreased kidney function on, 62t
Low-molecular-weight heparins
  for critically ill with kidney disease, 64
  decreased kidney function on, 60t

M

Machine alarms, on fluid management, 42
Magnesium
  functions of, 196
  plasma, clinical symptoms and, 197, 197t

therapeutic applications of, 197–198
Magnesium disorders
  in critically ill, 196–198
  clinical manifestations of, 189t
  differential diagnosis of, 191t
  hypermagnesemia, 189t, 191t, 197–198, 197t
  hypomagnesemia, 189t, 191t, 196–197
  management of, 189t
  hypermagnesemia, 197–198, 197t
  clinical manifestations of, 189t, 197
  differential diagnosis of, 191t
  management of, 189t, 197
  hypomagnesemia, 196–197
  causes of, 196
  clinical manifestations of, 189t, 196
  differential diagnosis of, 191t
  management of, 189t, 197
  after renal transplant, 146–148, 147t
Malnutrition, in critically ill
  assessment of, 202–203, 204t
  stages of, 203t
Mannitol, for AKI prevention in shock, 53
MDRD equation, 99
Medium-chain fatty acids, 207
Membranoproliferative glomerulonephritis (MPGN), in children, 122
Meperidine, 64, 65t
Metabolic acidosis, 132–134, 132t
  renal replacement therapy for, 72, 134
Metabolic alkalosis, 132t, 134–135
Metabolism, drug, 58
Metformin
  with chronic kidney disease, 32
  lactic acidosis with, 165–166
Methanol poisoning, renal replacement therapy for, 73t
Metolazone
  dosing of, 71t
  for volume overload, 70–71
Micronutrient requirements, 207
Midazolam, 65t, 66

Middle molecules, 88
Midodrine, 103t, 104
Morphine
    for critically ill with kidney
        disease, 64, 65t
    decreased kidney function
        on, 63t
Multicystic dysplastic kidney
    (MCDK), 124–125
Multiple organ dysfunction
    (MODS), 88
Muromonab-CD3, 154t
Mycophenolate mofetil, 153t
Mycophenolic acid, 153t
Myxedema coma, 173–174

N

N-acetyl-cysteine (NAC),
    for AKI prevention in
    shock, 53
Nadolol
    for critically ill with kidney
        disease, 66
    decreased kidney function
        on, 62t
Neomycin, 33
Nephrin, 126
Nephritis
    acute tubulointerstitial
        AKI in, 16–17
    in children, 123
    interstitial, AKI management
        in, 8
Nephronophthisis (NPHP),
    125
Nephrotic syndrome, in
    children
    congenital nephrotic
        syndrome, 126–127
    idiopathic nephrotic
        syndrome, 125–126
Nephrotoxins. See also specific
    types
    acute kidney injury from,
        6, 7t
    avoidance of, with chronic
        kidney disease, 32–33
Neuromuscular blockade, with
    chronic kidney disease, 36
Neutrophil Gelatinase-
    Associated Lipocalin
    (NGAL), 99
NGAL, 99
Non–Shiga-toxin (Stx)–
    associated hemolytic-
    uremic syndrome, AKI in,
    19–20
Nonsteroidal anti-inflammatory
    drugs (NSAIDs)
    with chronic kidney disease,
        33

for critically ill with kidney
    disease, 64
Nonthyroidal illness
    syndrome, 174–175
Noradrenaline. See
    Norepinephrine
Norepinephrine (NE)
    for AKI prevention in shock,
        51, 51t
    for AKI with cirrhosis,
        103t, 104
Nothing per oral (NPO),
    204–205
Nutrient requirements, in
    critically ill, 205–207
    caloric, 205–206
    carbohydrate, 206
    lipid, 206–207
    micronutrients, 207
    protein, 206
Nutrition
    in critically ill, 201–208
    in burn patients, 207
    in elderly, 207
    interventions for, 201,
        204–205
    malnutrition in, 202–203,
        203t, 204t
    nutrient requirements in,
        205–207
    in obese, 207
    starvation, 201–202
    in trauma, 202, 207–208
    enteral, 204
    immunonutrition in, 205
    on RRT outcome, 85
    total parenteral, 205
Nutritional intervention (NI),
    201, 204–205

O

Obese, nutrition in, 207
Octreotide, for AKI with
    cirrhosis, 103t, 104
Off-time
    definition of, 41
    potential problems in, 41–42
Oliguria, 3
Omega-3 fatty acids, 207
Omega-6 fatty acids, 207
Opiates, 64, 65t
Oral intake, 204
Overload, fluid, 39
Oxidative stress, in combined
    kidney-lung failure, 93

P

Paraganglioma, in children, 129
Passive leg raising (PLR), 44–45
Patient fluid balance, 39

Peak concentration
    hypothesis, 89
Pediatrics, renal disorders in,
    119–130
    acute glomerulonephritis,
        121–123
    poststreptococcal, 121–122
    rapidly progressive,
        122–123
    congenital disorders of the
        kidney, 123–125
    hydronephrosis, 123
    multicystic dysplastic
        kidney, 124–125
    nephronophthisis, 125
    posterior urethral valves,
        124
    prune belly syndrome, 124
    ureteropelvic junction
        obstruction, 124
    hemolytic uremic syndrome,
        119–121
    D- HUS (atypical HUS),
        120–121
    D+ HUS (typical HUS),
        119–120
    hypertension, 127–130
    blood pressure
        measurements in, 128
    coarctation of the aorta in,
        128–129
    hypertensive urgencies and
        emergencies in, 130
    pheochromocytoma or
        paraganglioma in, 129
    renal artery stenosis in, 128
    renal parenchymal disease
        in, 129
    nephrotic syndrome,
        125–127
    congenital, 126–127
    idiopathic, 125–126
Penicillins, 61t
Peritoneal dialysis, in
    pregnancy, 111
Pharmacokinetics, in kidney
    disease, 57–63. See also
    specific drugs
    absorption in, 57–58
    distribution in, 58
    excretion in, 59, 63, 65t
    metabolism in, 58
    for selected drugs, 60t–63t
Pharmacologic therapy, for
    AKI prevention in shock,
    49–55
    diuretics, 53–55
    mannitol, 53
    N-acetyl-cysteine, 53
    vasodilators and atrial
        natriuretic peptide,
        52–53

vasopressors and inotropes, 50–52, 50–51t
volume expansion, 49–50
Phenylephrine, 51t
Phenytoin
for critically ill with kidney disease, 66
decreased kidney function on, 63t
Pheochromocytoma, in children, 129
Phosphate
for diabetic ketoacidosis, 165
function of, 194
for hyperglycemic hyperosmolar coma, 165
Phosphatonins, 195
Phosphorus disorders
in critically ill, 194–195
clinical manifestations of, 188t–189t
differential diagnosis of, 191t
hyperphosphatemia, 188t–189t, 194–195
hypophosphatemia, 188t–189t, 191t, 194
management of, 188t–189t
pseudohyperphosphatemia, 195–196
after renal transplant, 146–148, 147t
hyperphosphatemia, 194–195
causes of, 194
clinical manifestations of, 188t–189t, 195
definition of, 195
differential diagnosis of, 191t
hypocalcemia with, 186
management of, 188t–189t, 195
after renal transplant, 146–148, 147t
hypophosphatemia, 194
clinical manifestations of, 188t, 194
differential diagnosis of, 191t
hypocalcemia with, 186
management of, 188t, 194
after renal transplant, 146–148, 147t
Pituitary adenomas, ACTH-secreting, 180
Placental abruption, 115t
Placenta previa, 115t
Plasma filtration coupled with adsorption (CPFA), 89
Pneumonia, in pregnancy, 116

Polymyxin B, 90
Positive-pressure ventilation, left-ventricular output in, 44–45, 45t
Posterior urethral valves (PUV), 124
Postoperative acute kidney injury, 6
Postpartum hemorrhage, 115t
Poststreptococcal glomerulonephritis (PSGN), in children, 121–122
Potassium, for diabetic ketoacidosis, 163t, 165
Potassium disorders
hyperkalemia, 141–142
management of, initial, 71–72
renal replacement therapy for, 71–72, 76
after renal transplant, 146–148, 146t
risks of, 71
signs of, 71
hypokalemia, 141–142
in diabetic, 165
after renal transplant, 146–148, 147t
Prednisone, for renal transplantation, 153t
Preeclampsia, 111–112, 112t, 113t
Pregnancy
hemorrhage in, 114, 115t
renal adaptations in
anatomic changes in, 107–108
infections in, 114–116
physiologic changes in, 108–109, 108t
renal disorders in, 107–117
amniotic fluid embolus in, 116
categories of, 107
causes of, non–pregnancy-specific, 116–117
definitions in, 107
diagnostic criteria for, 107
evaluation of, 109–110
hypertensive disorders of pregnancy in, 111–114 (See also Hypertensive disorders of pregnancy)
infections in, 114–116
management principles in, 110–111
obstruction in, 116
volume depletion in, 114, 115t
Pregnancy-related AKI. See Pregnancy, renal disorders in

Primary adrenal insufficiency, 177–179
Primary aldosteronism, 181–182
Primary glomerulonephritis, in children, 122
Procainamide, 65t
Propofol, 66
Propoxyphene, 64, 65t
Propranolol
for critically ill with kidney disease, 66
decreased kidney function on, 62t
Protein intake, in chronic kidney disease, 36
Protein requirements, 206
Proton-pump inhibitors (PPIs), 66
Prune belly syndrome, 124
Pseudohyperphosphatemia, 195–196
Pulmonary hypertension, after renal transplant, 145–146
Pyelonephritis, in pregnancy, 114

R

Radiocontrast agents
acute kidney injury from, 6, 7t, 13–16
epidemiology of, 13
pathophysiology of, 14
prevention strategies for, 14–16
risk factors for, 14
chronic kidney disease from, 31–32
renal replacement therapy for, 72–73, 74t
Rapidly progressive glomerulonephritis (RPGN), in children, 122–123
Rebound phenomenon, renal replacement therapy and, 72
Recessive familial nephrotic syndrome, 126–127
Relative adrenal insufficiency (RAI), 178–180
Renal artery stenosis, in children, 128
Renal failure. See also specific types
clinical manifestations of, 3
definition of, 3
manifestations of, 69, 70t

Renal function assessment, in liver disease, 97–100, 98t
  ancillary testing in, 99–100
  creatine based equations in, 99
  glomerular filtration rate in, 97, 98t
  serum creatine in, 98t, 99
Renal parenchymal disease, in children, 129
Renal replacement therapy (RRT), 69–76. *See also specific types*
  for acid-base disorders, 132
  for azotemia, 71
  for contrast agent toxicity, 72–73, 74t
  for cytokines, 74
  for drug and toxin removal, 72, 73t
  with hypercalcemia, 193
  for hyperkalemia, 71–72
  for metabolic acidosis, 72, 134
  "nonrenal" indications for, 72–74, 73t
  patient selection for, 75–76
  renal indications for, 69–72
  for sepsis and severe sepsis, 26–27, 88–90
  timing of, 74–75, 75t
  for volume overload, 69–70
Renal replacement therapy (RRT), in AKI, 8–9, 77–90
  arterio-venous *vs.* veno-venous blood circuits in, 79
  with cirrhosis, 105
  comparison of, 83
  dose of, recent randomized controlled trials on, 83–85, 84f, 85t
  epidemiology of, in-hospital, 77
  hemadsorption in, 89
  hemodynamic stability in, 85–88
  in continuous renal replacement therapy, 85
  fluid overload and mortality in, 87, 87f
  in intermittent hemodialysis, 86–87
  hemofiltration in
  high-volume, 89
  of large molecules, 88–90
  ideal treatment modality for, ICU, 77, 77t
  indications for, 78t
  modality choice in, 78–82, 78t
  advantages and disadvantages of, 79, 79t

considerations and components in, 78t
  convection and diffusion in, 82
  convective treatments in, 81–82
  definitions and nomenclature in, 79, 80f, 81–82
  indications in, 78t
  issues in, 80
  sustained low-efficiency dialysis in, 80–81
  nutrition on outcome in, 85
  plasma filtration coupled with hemadsorption in, 89
Renal transplantation, ICU management of, 143–155
  for bleeding/hypercoagulable state, 148
  for cardiovascular disease, 145, 145t
  for delayed or slow graft function, 143, 144t
  for hypertension, 149, 150t
  for infections, 148–149, 149f
  need for, 143
  for pulmonary hypertension, 145–146
  transplant medications in, 150–151, 150t–155t
  antibody preparations, 154t–155t
  antimetabolites, 153t
  calcineurin inhibitors, 152t
  drug-drug interactions of, 150t–151t
  steroids, 153t
  for volume/electrolyte abnormalities, 146–148, 146t–147t
Renal transplantation, prevalence of, 143
Renovascular disorders, acute kidney injury from, 6
Respiratory acidosis, 132t, 135–136
Respiratory alkalosis, 132t, 135–136
Resuscitation, initial, with chronic kidney disease, 35
Rhabdomyolysis, acute kidney injury from, 6
RIFLE classification, 3–4, 4f
Rituximab, 155t

S

Salicylate poisoning, renal replacement therapy for, 73t

Secondary adrenal insufficiency, 179–180
Sedation, 36
Sedatives, for critically ill with kidney disease, 66
Sepsis, 23–27
  acute kidney injury in, 5
  epidemiology of, 23
  volume resuscitation in, 23–25, 24f
  renal replacement therapy for, 26–27
  severe
    continuous renal replacement therapy for, 89
    endotoxin in, 89–90
    multiple organ dysfunction from, 88
    water-soluble mediators in, 88
  vasoconstrictors in, 25–26
Septic abortion, 114
Septic shock
  continuous renal replacement therapy for, 89
  endotoxin in, 89–90
  management of, AKI and, 23–26
  arginine vasopressin for, 25–26
  catecholamines for, 25–26
  corticosteroids for, 26
  dopamine for, 25
  epinephrine for, 25
  vasopressin for, 25–26
  volume resuscitation for, 23–25, 24f
  multiple organ dysfunction from, 88
  water-soluble mediators in, 88
Serum creatine assessment, 98t, 99
Serum cystatin C, 98t
Severe sepsis
  continuous renal replacement therapy for, 89
  endotoxin in, 89–90
  water-soluble mediators in, 88
Shiga-toxin (Stx)–associated hemolytic-uremic syndrome, AKI in, 18–20
Shock, septic
  continuous renal replacement therapy for, 89
  endotoxin in, 89–90
  multiple organ dysfunction from, 88

water-soluble mediators in, 88
Shock management
preventing acute kidney injury in, 49–55
diuretics in, 53–55
mannitol in, 53
N-acetyl-cysteine in, 53
vasodilators and atrial natriuretic peptide in, 52–53
vasopressors and inotropes in, 50–52, 50–51t
volume expansion in, 49–50
in septic shock, 23–26
arginine vasopressin in, 25–26
catecholamines in, 25–26
corticosteroids in, 26
dopamine in, 25
epinephrine in, 25
vasopressin in, 25–26
volume resuscitation in, 23–25, 24f
Short-chain fatty acids, 206
Sirolimus, 152t
Slow graft function (SGF), renal, 143, 144t
Solumedrol, 153t
Sotalol
for critically ill with kidney disease, 66
decreased kidney function on, 62t
Spironolactone, 32
Spontaneous abortion, 115t
Starvation
controlled, 204–205
pathogenesis of, 201
physiologic adaptation to, 201–202
Steroids
for renal transplantation, 153t
for septic shock, 26
Steroid sensitive nephrotic syndrome, 125–126
Stress ulcer prophylaxis, with chronic kidney disease, 35
Surviving Sepsis Campaign, 24
Sustained low-efficiency dialysis (SLED), 80–81
Syndrome of inappropriate ADH secretion (SIADH), 139–141

T

T3, 171
T4, 171
Tacrolimus, 152t
Terlipressing

for AKI prevention in shock, 51
for AKI with cirrhosis, 103t, 104
Theophylline
for AKI prevention in shock, 53
poisoning with, renal replacement therapy for, 73t
Thiazide diuretics
for critically ill with kidney disease, 66
decreased kidney function on, 63t
dosing of, 71t
for volume overload, 70–71
Thrombin inhibitors
for critically ill with kidney disease, 64
decreased kidney function on, 60t
Thrombotic thrombocytopenic purpura (TTP), in pregnancy, 112–113, 113t
Thymoglobulin, 154t
Thyroid conditions, 171–175
hyperthyroidism, 172
hypothyroidism, 171–172
myxedema coma, 173–174
nonthyroidal illness syndrome, 174–175
pathogenesis of, 171
prevalence of, 171
thyroid storm, 172–173
Thyroid storm, 172–173
Tinzaparin
for critically ill with kidney disease, 64
decreased kidney function on, 60t
Torsemide dosing, 71t
Total parenteral nutrition (TPN), 205
Toxin removal. See also specific toxins
renal replacement therapy for, 72, 73t
Transjugular intrahepatic porto-systemic shunt (TIPS), 104
Transplantation
liver, for AKI with cirrhosis, 105, 105t
renal, ICU management of, 143–155 (See also Renal transplantation, ICU management of)
Trauma, nutrition in, 202, 207–208
Troponins, cardiac, 32

Trousseau's sign, 186
Tubulointerstitial nephritis, acute, 16–17, 123

U

Ulcer prophylaxis, with chronic kidney disease, 35
Uremic syndrome
clinical manifestations of, 70t
pathogenesis of, 71
Ureteropelvic junction obstruction, 124
Urinary creatine clearance, 98t
Urinary tract obstruction, in pregnancy, 116

V

Valproic acid poisoning, renal replacement therapy for, 73t
Vancomycin
with chronic kidney disease, 33
for critically ill with kidney disease, 60t–61t, 65
decreased kidney function on, 61t
Vascular occlusion test (VOT), tissue O2 saturation changes in, 43–44
Vasculitis, in children, 122
Vasoconstrictors
for AKI prevention in shock, 51–52, 50t
for AKI with cirrhosis, 103–104, 103t
for sepsis, 25–26
Vasodilators. See also specific types
for AKI prevention in shock, 52–53
Vasopressin
for AKI prevention in shock, 51
for AKI with cirrhosis, 103t, 104
for septic shock, 25–26
Vasopressors, for AKI prevention in shock, 50–52, 50–51t
Veno-venous blood circuits, 79
Viral infections, after renal transplantation, 148–149, 149f
Vitamin C, 207
Volume depletion, in pregnancy, 114, 115t
Volume disorders, after renal transplant, 146–148

Volume expansion, for AKI
    prevention in shock,
    49–50
Volume overload
    diuretics for, 70
    pathogenesis of, 69
    renal replacement therapy
        for, 69–70, 76
Volume-responsive acute
    kidney injury, 5
Volume responsiveness
    definition of, 44

left-ventricular output
    in positive-pressure
        ventilation in, 44–45, 45t
    passive leg raising in, 44–45,
        45t
Volume resuscitation, for
    septic shock, 23–25, 24f
Voriconazole
    for critically ill with kidney
        disease, 60t–61t, 65
    decreased kidney function
        on, 61t

W

Warfarin, 60t
Waterhouse–Friderichsen
    syndrome, 178

Z

Zona fasciculata, 177
Zona glomerulosa, 177
Zona reticularis, 177